7-85

# Studies in Everyday Medical Life

MEDICINE IN SOCIETY SERIES
*General Editors:* Malcolm Johnson, Una Maclean and Peter Sheldrake

**APPROACHES TO ILLNESS**
Robert Dingwall

# Studies in Everyday Medical Life

*edited by Michael Wadsworth and David Robinson*

MARTIN ROBERTSON

616
S 933

First published in 1976 by Martin Robertson & Co. Ltd., 17 Quick Street, London N1 8HL

ISBN 0 85520 147 9

Typeset by Preface Graphics Ltd., Salisbury.
Reproduced, printed by photolithography and bound at the Pitman Press, Bath.

# Contents

# Contributors

ELIZABETH M. ANDERSON     Institute of Education, Thomas Coram Research Unit, University of London.

MICHAEL BLOOR     Medical Research Council, Institute of Medical Sociology, University of Aberdeen.

MALCOLM COULTHARD and MARGARET ASHBY     Department of English Language and Literature, English Language Research Unit, University of Birmingham.

ALAN DAVIS and PHILIP STRONG     Medical Research Council, Institute of Medical Sociology, University of Aberdeen.

ROBERT DINGWALL     Medical Research Council, Institute of Medical Sociology, University of Aberdeen.

NIGEL GOLDIE     Department of Sociology, Polytechnic of the South Bank, London.

DAVID INGLEBY     Medical Research Council Unit on Environmental Factors in Mental and Physical Illness, London School of Economics.

DAVID ROBINSON     Addiction Research Unit, Institute of Psychiatry, University of London.

JOANNA RYAN     Unit for Research on Medical Applications of Psychology, University of Cambridge.

GERRY STIMSON     Addiction Research Unit, Institute of Psychiatry, University of London.

MICHAEL WADSWORTH — Medical Research Council Unit on Environmental Factors in Mental and Physical Illness, London School of Economics.

BARBARA WEBB — Medical Sociology Research Centre, University College of Swansea.

PATRICK WEST — Department of Child Health, University of Bristol.

In addition to the contributors to this volume, the seminar benefited greatly from the participation of Diana Burfield, Richard Compton, Elizabeth Cooper, Anthony Costello, Heather Gibson, John Harvard-Watts, Margaret Voysey, Peter Whittingham and Sharon Williams.

# Preface

The essays in this book are all in some way concerned with everyday life in medical settings. They were prepared for a seminar held at the London School of Economics which grew out of a quiet bar side conversation during the final plenary session of a medical sociology conference some months earlier. It was clear that the contributions that had stimulated us most were not the papers asking 'Whither Medical Sociology?' or the pieces on grand medical—organisational theory, or the thinly veiled policy statements, or the plaintive cries from the heart of those attempting to teach sociology to medical students, but rather the reports from those who were attempting to understand the nitty-gritty of everyday medical life. It seemed a good idea, therefore, to bring together some of these people to present and discuss their work.

Our aim was not to construct 'a representative sample of British sociologists and psychologists' but rather to bring together some of the people who we knew to be doing work in the particular research area that interested us. There is no way, therefore, in which this volume can be said to present a systematic coverage of everyday medical life. For example, at the most obvious level, while there are essays that focus on the career of the patient, there are none on the career of the doctor. Similarly, while there are discussions of doctor—patient communication and patient—patient communication, there are none on doctor—doctor communication. The contributions are linked together merely by the authors' common concern to tease out the ground rules of certain medical encounters and situations.

This has been a collaborative venture. We, as organisers, merely provided the basic minimum of administrative support necessary to enable a small number of people from England, Scotland and Wales to come together and discuss their studies of 'everyday medical life'. If that exercise was of any value to the participants, and if readers find something of interest in this volume, then it is only because people produced and circulated their papers well before the meeting, contributed fully to discussion in the meeting, made detailed written comments on other people's papers after the meeting, and revised their own before publication deadlines.

We are particularly grateful for editorial help from Mary Squires and Serena Dalrymple.

*Michael Wadsworth*
*David Robinson*

ACKNOWLEDGEMENT

Permission was generously granted to reproduce material in Chapter 7 from *Going to See the Doctor: the consultation process in general practice*, © Gerry Stimson and Barbara Webb, Routledge and Kegan Paul, London, 1975, and in Chapter 9 from *From Drinking to Alcoholism: a sociological commentary*, David Robinson, © John Wiley and Sons, London, 1976. The editors of *Sociological Review* generously gave permission to include, as Chapter 6, a revised version of Accomplishing Profession © Robert Dingwall, *Sociological Review* 24.2. 331—349, 1976.

# Introduction

A great deal of the research done by social scientists in relation to medicine could be called 'service research'. That is, it sets out to answer questions usually posed by medical practitioners and administrators, and therefore geared to explaining or reducing particular health problems, easing the clinical task or making more efficient the organisation and delivery of medical care. Rather less research is concerned to ask why certain things are assumed in the ordinary everyday practice of medicine to be health 'problems', what is involved in the routine activity of a 'clinical task' or what counts as being 'efficient'. This book examines some of the assumptions and definitions of everyday life in medical settings. It illustrates the diversity of ways in which social scientists are thinking about a great many areas of contemporary life, not merely medicine.

Over the past thirty years there have been three major types of social science research in relation to medicine. First, there have been the administrative—organisational studies concerned with the distribution and use of services and manpower, and with the formulation and efficacy of policy. Closely related to these, social—epidemiological studies have set out to investigate the role of various aspects of the social environment in the aetiology and management of illness conditions, disability and handicap. The third set of studies, by contrast, rather than concentrating on organisations and particular illness conditions, have attempted to assess the meaning of illness for the individual in terms of family and other social obligations. These 'illness behaviour' studies have emphasised the importance of the social context in which illness is experienced and responded to.

This book grows naturally from these concerns. The emphasis is on everyday life in *particular* medical settings, since it is only on the basis of detailed knowledge of this kind that general statements can be made about medical organisations, medical practice and the experience of health and illness. The essays range from the linguistic analysis of a medical consultation to discussions of professional ideology, while two concentrate on the question of 'accounts'. Webb and Stimson (chapter 7) focus on the 'stories' that people tell of their encounters with professionals and show how this story-telling is a routine part of the process by which people not only make sense of the past but also attempt to redress the inequalities between the lay and the medical world. Davis and Strong (chapter 8) concentrate on the accounts that physiotherapists and occupational therapists give of their 'work' in their attempts to build on children's taken-for-granted understanding of 'play' and transform it into the kind of activity that is demanded by the therapeutic regime.

Three of the chapters deal in some way with the question of communication between doctors and their patients. Wadsworth (chapter 1), after noting that surprisingly little research has been done on consulting-room interactions, reviews such work as there is, and draws our attention to the need for detailed analyses which do not take for granted at the outset what is to count as 'successful' or 'effective' communication, but which aim rather to investigate the rules, routines and procedures in terms of which patients and doctors organise their everyday consultations. Coulthard and Ashby (chapter 5) have used doctor—patient interviews as one of four 'socially defined situations' in which to try to discover how people produce and interpret coherent discourse according to general linguistic rules and structures. They outline some of the basic categories of a linguistic model of discourse and characterise some of the typical linguistic units through which doctor—patient communication is realised. Bloor (chapter 4), on the other hand, takes the linguistic rules for granted and, on the basis of systematic observation of ENT clinic consultations, focuses on the question of how specialists' investigating routines may facilitate 'specialist autonomy'.

Anderson and West are both concerned with patient careers. In chapter 3 Anderson examines the relationship between doctors and the mothers of physically handicapped children at the time when the decision about school placement is being made. West (chapter 2) analyses the process by which a child who has had a seizure becomes defined as an epileptic. For various reasons the physician is often unwilling to name the disorder and provide a framework in terms of which parents can understand and cope with the situation. Over time, however, the doctor is increasingly challenged about diagnosis and other medical decisions and, as a result, has to 'work' hard to maintain his claim to competence.

Dingwall (chapter 6) discusses the literature on health professions, and in particular questions the 'attribute' approach which assumes that it is possible to draw up a list of fixed criteria for recognising 'a profession' and on which there will be general consensus. He describes aspects of his own work on health visitors, which is informed by a perspective which takes 'profession' as a matter to be 'accomplished' in everyday interaction. In the other chapter that focuses particularly on professional activity, Robinson (chapter 9) looks at referrals to an out-patient department and at the question of how referrals, once made, are handled by the hospital staff. Based on case notes, records and the correspondence between various types of referral agent and the hospital, an attempt is made to explain why some referrals are accepted and others not, and how 'uncontrollable' or 'unrefusable' referrals are discouraged.

The final set of essays deals with the definition and handling of mental illness. Ryan (chapter 10) presents a critique of present views on subnormality and outlines the historical, political and medical attitudes that underpin present policy. She discusses the extremely complex question of how the psychology, both pure and applied, that is done in relation to subnormality reflects and reinforces certain ideological assumptions about the place of the inept in our society. The various activities of psychologists, she claims, such as diagnosis, assessment, research and behaviour modification, all play their part in the social processes that create and maintain so many people as stupid. In chapter 11 Goldie discusses how psychiatrists justify control over the treatment of what they take to be mental illness and how they view their own activities and those of their non-psychiatric colleagues. The diffuseness of the mandate that psychiatrists claim for themselves enables them to set the terms on which other staff have access to patients. In the final chapter Ingleby argues that what we construe as mental illnesses are, if we examine them closely, manifestations of our culture and way of life and, further, that we seek to treat these manifestations as person-centred illnesses only because of the constraints inherent in the concept of 'welfare'.

The contributions in this volume are grouped in terms of simple themes. But it will be clear from reading them that as many things divide essays in the same group as unite them. There was a suggestion at the end of the meeting that the introduction should contain some grand interdisciplinary theoretical structure which could in some way accommodate and indicate the nature of the relationships between the essays that follow. Although that was not the point of the exercise as we saw it, it was certainly open to any of the participants who felt so moved to attempt some integrative theory-building. If anyone had done so the piece would have been given a prominent place in this book. None appeared!

# Patient Careers
and Communication

# 1 Studies of Doctor–Patient Communication

## by Michael Wadsworth

Surprisingly few sociologists have studied doctor—patient consultations. Much effort has been invested in the study of why patients visit their doctors, and how they reach the decision to do so; into how well patients comply with doctors' advice and instructions, and into demonstrating the social complexity of the whole interlinked process. This makes it all the more surprising that the consultation at the conclusion of this process, the source of patients' future preconception of consultations, has received so little attention. It is particularly surprising in view of the accepted importance of communication between doctors and patients in the treatment of illness. In relation to chronic illness, Joyce *et al.* (1969), for example, say that 'in rheumatic and degenerative joint disease . . . communication is virtually the only form of treatment there is,' while Davis (1960) reported that

> . . . uncertainty, a *real* factor in the early diagnosis and treatment of the paralysed child, came more and more to serve the purely managerial ends of the treatment personnel in their interaction with parents. Long after the doctor himself was no longer in doubt about the outcome, the perpetuation of uncertainty in doctor-to-family communication, although perhaps neither premeditated nor intended, can nonetheless best be understood in terms of its functions in the treatment system.

Reasons for the paucity of good field studies of consultations are rooted not only in the traditional views of the confidentiality of the consulting room, but also in the complexity of the nature of such encounters, reflected in the many ways in which it might be studied. In a later chapter Coulthard and Ashby present work on the linguistic organisation of doctor—patient interviews. Others have considered the relative 'success' or 'failure' of consultations as seen,

3

for example, from the patient's point of view. This has sometimes taken the form of patients' expressions, after a consultation with the doctor, of how completely they felt they had been able to explain their symptoms and problems. Pratt *et al.* (1957), Siegel and Dillehay (1966) and Cartwright (1968) all report that doctors seem to assume too high an ability in patients to initiate discussion. Korsch and Negrete (1972) report that 'among the eight hundred mothers 26% told interviewers after the session with the doctor that they had not mentioned their greatest concern to the physician because they did not have an opportunity or were not encouraged to do so'. Joyce and his colleagues (1969) noted a reciprocal effect in that 'articulate patients made more importations. They were told more by the doctor, and told it more often. . . . They were also given a significantly better prognosis.' Ima, Tagliacozzo and Lashof (1970) found evidence that the way that the doctor 'categorised' the patient affected the kind of communication that took place. Some were more articulate than others, while private patients were less likely than clinic patients to be considered 'a problem patient'. 'Our data suggests a "syndrome" in which negative orientation towards clinic patients involves both a more negative view of clinic patients, and tendencies toward a firmer approach to problem patients.' On the other hand some investigators find that the patient's judgement of the doctor's friendliness and interest has an important effect on the outcome of the encounter. This also applies to the communication with the parents of child patients. 'When the doctor does express negative feelings, the mother is likely to be dissatisfied with the visit and fail to comply with his advice. Conversely, a substantial showing of positive affect by the doctor to the mother enhances her satisfaction and compliance.' (Korsch and Negrete, 1972.)

From the doctor's point of view success or failure of consultations has been judged in two ways: whether or not patients carried out instructions, and how well they remembered advice, instructions and the diagnosis. In investigating how well patients carried out their instructions Caron and Roth (1968) found that most doctors overestimated their patients' actual compliance with the treatment regime. In a study of how well patients remembered what their doctors said, Ley and Spelman (1965) reported evidence of selective recall. Patients tended to forget instructions and advice, and to recall diagnostic statements.

Discussion of what might account for these kinds of communication 'problems' usually refers to the patient's and doctor's views of one another at this consultation, views that have been built up from previous experience (Joyce *et al.*, 1969; Ima *et al.*, 1970). Differences between doctors and patients in respect of ethnic group, social class and educational background are also commonly put forward as explanations for communication problems. Shortage of the doctor's time is also given as an additional aggravating factor. Joyce *et al.* (1969) conclude that the doctor 'might consider carefully exactly what he wishes the patient to remember. He might engage the *patient* to write it down and keep a check that it has been registered correctly'. Without specifically recommending a course of action Ima and his colleagues (1970) merely suggest that 'the adjustment to the vast array of patients and their moral character is a source of difficulty for some physicians', while both Caron and Roth (1968) and Duff and Hollingshead (1968) implicate socioeconomic differences between doctors and patients in problems of communication. Cartwright (1966, p. 219) pointed out that the content of current medical school curricula tends to make general practitioners feel 'resentful' and 'fail to recognise an underlying need for help', when presented with what they take to be trivia. Thus, it is hardly surprising that Ford should conclude that the doctor . . .

. . . can work effectively with a patient who is well educated, self reliant, and responsive to treatment. Second, in terms of motivation, he reports that he can practice well and enlist the aid of others when the patient believes in him. Negatively, the patient hinders practice when he escapes control by being uncooperative, unresponsive to treatment, or hostile. [Ford *et al.*, 1967, p. 95.]

Nor is it surprising that most of the work on doctor—patient communications is concerned simply with content. After experimenting with dummy information and people posing as patients, Ley (1972), for example, concluded that 'the amount of recall can be increased by categorising the information presented and by presenting the information in short words and sentences'.

THE CONSULTATION

These rather circumscribed conclusions indicate an under-appreciation of the sociological work on doctor—patient relationships which, although not always specifically concerned with the consultation, contains many points that need to be taken into account in an understanding of consultations. Before drawing conclusions about 'success' or 'failure' of doctor—patient communication it is necessary to appreciate that the consultation is not a one way process in which patients simply come to ask for advice. Many studies have shown that patients come prepared with some idea as to what is wrong, whilst other patients seem less well prepared but equally in need of information as well as advice and treatment. In the study by Joyce *et al.* (1969) there were 'indications . . . that reassurance is of no value whatever to some patients since it is never registered'. Somewhat similarly, Korsch and Negrete (1972) note that 'some patients were so preoccupied with their dominant concern that they were unable to listen to the physician'. In the same study Korsch and Negrete show how parents of a child with a heart murmur are at some pains to discover the cause of the illness, and although they are given an explanation by the examining doctor they nevertheless put forward their thoughts about causation for appraisal. Balint (1957) has also observed, from many years of clinical experience, that for the patient 'the need to understand is so compelling that it may actually outdo the desire to be cured' (p. 280). Similarly the tendency noticed by Ley and Spelman (1965) for patients to recall the diagnosis better than the advice seems to indicate a desire for understanding.

It is also important to note that the consultation is rarely an isolated event, even within the current episode of illness. In the next chapter Patrick West shows the very considerable effect on doctor—patient communication of the change in relationships that takes place during the course of a long-term illness requiring many consultations, even with different doctors. His work illustrates changes over time in both patients' ideas of the nature of their illness and its treatment, and in their response to how doctors typically 'handle' or 'manage' the consultation itself.

It is in the management of the consultation that the differences of the immediate objectives or agendas of the doctor and the patient are best observed. In their study of tape recordings and transcripts of real life consultations Korsch and Negrete (1972) give an example of how the doctor must, whilst he is in the process of making a diagnosis, answer questions from the patient's parents, and give an explanation of the condition and its causes. It looks as if it is this mix of activities that leads him to explain the prognosis for the child in highly technical language. For example, when the mother asks what might have caused the hole in the child's heart, the doctor gives an explanation, and concludes that it is 'one thing that they never get SBE from . . . it's the only heart lesion in which they don't'. In the same study, it is also evident that although they receive several explanations and advice in such technical language, which they are very unlikely to have understood, apparently the parents do not press the doctor for further elaboration. This kind of assumed inequality of opportunity to put questions and to pursue points of concern, and the way in which such inequality may be redressed, are discussed elsewhere in this volume.

It is clear that the relatively few studies of the consultation confirm the inferences that may be made from other studies of particular points in time during the whole process of a consultation, that doctors and patients seem very often to conduct their communications with different immediate ends in mind. To see why this should be so it is helpful to look for possible explanations among the sociological and other work on pre-consultation behaviour, to see the consultation as part of the patient's progression from his first recognition of ill health through to a medical diagnosis, rather than allowing ourselves to be misled by seeing the consultation as an isolated incident. It is then much more likely that more practical conclusions may be drawn than observation about the importance of class and ethnic differences between doctors and patients, which are hardly likely to be very helpful in training health care professionals. That communication is important is self-evident not only because of the need for comprehension of the doctor's advice and instructions, but also because, particularly in chronic illness, it may itself be at least an important part of the treatment, and at most constitute the treatment itself.

THE PATIENT'S VIEW

There are two kinds of reasons to expect a difference in objective between patients and doctors at consultations. Firstly, as part of the process of accommodating to sickness experience the potential patient assesses the reasons for and implications of his complaints. As Robinson (1971) points out, this assessment will by no means be 'objective', and will be closely related to his social and psychological circumstances at the time. 'Questions of health and illness were always considered in conjunction with assessments of *current* ideas, demands and beliefs about appropriate ways of behaving. It was mentioned ... that Mrs B obviously considered it perfectly consistent to say that she was "very healthy" and yet to be waiting to be called into hospital for a heart operation' (p. 116). Certainly, there would usually be plenty of time before the consultation during which to consider the nature of the complaints experienced. I have discussed elsewhere (Wadsworth, 1974) the reasons for thinking that people accommodate to sickness experience and gradually change their norms of what constitutes 'good health' for them.

The potential patient will also consider the possible consequences for his future life of being 'labelled' as a sufferer from a particular disease. If he has a feeling that the complaint may be in some way attributable to his way of life, or his mismanagement of it as perceived by commonly accepted medical standards, then the patient's preconception and his management of the desired outcome of the consultation will be different from that of the patient who has a condition which is widely accepted as beyond his influence. Contrast, for example, the difference in reaction of workmates and family to the case of the young man hospitalised, or otherwise clearly labelled as having a disease often said to be associated with stress, such as a peptic ulcer, with the reaction to another man of the same age who has to have his appendix removed. There is a growing awareness, particularly through health education campaigns, of the part the individual may play in the genesis of his illness. There is plenty of epidemiological evidence to show that these 'stress' illnesses are increasing in the western urbanised world.

Stoetzel (1960) hypothesises that, through the diffusion of psychomatic theories, our society may return, after the guilt-free germ theories, to a self-blaming conception of illness in which the individual feels himself responsible for his illness because of the mental conflicts that have induced it, while in Balint's work the idea of the participation of the individual in the genesis of his illness finds particularly clear expression.

Zola (1972) presents evidence of a feeling of responsibility for self-involvement illness in an experiment with undergraduate students:

> I asked a class of forty undergraduates, mostly 17, 18 and 19, to recall the last time they were sick, disabled or hurt and to then

record how they did or would have communicated this experience to a child under the age of five. . . . The opening words of the sick, injured, person to the query of the child were

'I feel bad'.

Zola found that the reply of the child was inevitable: 'What did you do wrong?' The 'ill person' in no case corrected the child's perspective but rather joined it at that level.

On bacteria

'There are good germs and bad germs and sometimes the bad germs. . . .'

On catching a cold

'Well you know sometimes when your mother says, "Wrap up or be careful or you'll catch a cold", well I . . . If you are good and do all the things the Dr and your mother tell you, you will get better.'

Not only will many people have considered their present involvement in their complaints and the effects of these complaints on their future lives, but also, since an increasing proportion of illness has a gradual and insidious onset, they would have had plenty of time to become accustomed to them, and this too has an important effect.

Thus, the individual will come to the consultation prepared with some sort of view of his involvement in the illness, some concept of what the illness may be, and some hopes and fears about its possible personal and social consequences. In addition he may well have preconceived ideas about the doctor and how to manage the consultation, as is discussed elsewhere in this book by Webb and Stimson.

## THE DOCTOR'S VIEW

The doctor on the other hand approaches the consultation from a very different standpoint. Before he can give advice about the management of the illness or give a prognosis he must first make a diagnosis. In their book entitled *The Future General Practitioner* a team from the Royal College of General Practitioners (1972) explain how a doctor makes a diagnosis: 'He will thus record, in his mind or in writing, a pattern which can be compared with patterns in a text book or remembered from previous clinical experience. From these the one most closely resembling the present case is chosen. This process of selection and matching results in a label — the diagnosis' (p. 16).

The doctor seems at the consultation to be taking all the information presented to him by the patient, or gleaned by him from the patient, and subjecting it to a process of reduction, in order to test for goodness of fit with pre-established models of illnesses. As Susser (1973) says,

> . . . the causes of disease sought by a medical scientist are limited by his concept of disease and by his frame of reference. . . . To choose a frame of reference is to choose a limited set of causal relationships within an ecological system. The choice is the outcome of the needs and consciousness of an investigator in a particular situation but on logical grounds it is an arbitrary procedure. The specificity of one to one relationships can only be attained by such arbitrary procedures. [pp. 42—3]

Thus it seems clear that the doctor must operate by taking the most likely clues that the consultation throws up, so that once he feels that he is 'on to something' he is likely to pay particular attention to checking out all the points of his frame of reference with the patient. This may sometimes explain why the doctor seems in relentless pursuit of a point which seems disruptive to the patient's view of things. The doctor's objective is, pragmatically, to come to a decision about the cause of the symptoms that are presented, and his task is to bring order through the process of diagnosis. He must reduce the information that is offered to him and seek out further information in accordance with a frame of reference he had in mind; namely, the diagnosis pattern of the illness from which he thinks the patient suffers. It is significant that Balint (1957) called the pre-consultation phase 'unorganised' illness.

DOCTOR—PATIENT COMMUNICATION

Perhaps, after all, it is not surprising that the majority of studies in this area seem to draw conclusions that bear little relationship to the reality of everyday life. It is, for example, hardly likely that asking doctors or teaching medical students to speak to their patients in a particular way will have much effect, if the origin of the problem lies in the very considerable differences in approach that doctors and patients bring to a consultation. Although explanations in terms of ethnic or social class differences between patients and doctors may well explain parts of the problem, they bear very little relationship to the situation in everyday life, and are certainly much too compressed as theoretical concepts from or on which to build working dynamic hypotheses. In the opening chapter of his book *Understanding Everyday Life*, Douglas (1971) writes that:

> . . . all of these arguments against the basic proposition that *all* of the *science* of sociology *necessarily* begins with the understanding of everyday life share one simple but fundamental failure. They have all failed to follow their empirical evidence (or what they purport to be empirical evidence) back to its actual source. Whenever we do this we find that there is only one source of empirical evidence for all of sociology (once we agree that social meanings are necessarily a form of evidence we are going to use in our theories). And that source is our understanding of everyday life. [p. 5]

The field of psychological and sociological studies of communication in medical situations is in need of more investigations that base their empirical evidence in everyday life situations. Such studies are required both for theoretical and practical reasons. They would provide a starting point for hypothesising about communications between doctors and patients. They would not begin with a view to drawing conclusions that would be statistically extrapolatable to the whole of the universe of communications between doctors and patients, but would be concerned with investigating the whole universe of what goes on at a consultation. Nor will they begin with preconceptions of success and failure of doctor—patient communications, for clearly, if the participants do not have identical objectives, then success and failure are to be seen as relative terms. These studies will set out to investigate the rules, routines and procedures that doctors and patients use to organise consultations, and their conclusions will be referrable to everyday life situations in a way that present studies in this field are not.

This chapter has attempted to show that there is a need to build on earlier work on communication, to follow-up leads given by this work, and to turn now to more detailed and observational kinds of methods. It is suggested that there is a need to avoid conforming to statistical requirements too early, at the conceptual stage of research, otherwise useful study data may ultimately be so reduced for the purposes of analysis that they can no longer be usefully interpreted when they have been analysed. There is also a need to avoid building working hypotheses on theoretical sociological constructs rather than on observation of what is happening all around us, in everyday life.

# 2  The Physician and the Management of Childhood Epilepsy

## by Patrick West

I gotta go all down the doctors to get some tablets to let him think she was still taking them. I was ashamed not to go down to get the, you know, new tablets. [Mother of epileptic daughter who followed this routine for five years]

Rule 4 — The obligation — to seek technically competent help, namely, in the most usual case, that of a physician and to co-operate with him in the process of trying to get well. [T. Parsons, 1951, on the sick role]

This chapter examines the position of the physician as a key 'significant other' in the process by which a child who has had some kind of seizure becomes defined as epileptic. The aim of the investigation is to treat this process in terms of a 'career' with specific consequences for the labelled person and others with whom he interacts (Becker, 1963; Goffman, 1963, 1968).[1] The doctor, in this general formulation, is evidently one important actor to be considered, since it is assumed that the social construction of illness and its meaning for the patient and others is almost entirely determined by the medical profession (Freidson, 1970).

The significance ascribed to the physician in this perspective would appear to depend upon the existence of fairly well defined rules of diagnosis and patient management. It seems logical that there should be relative agreement within the medical profession about the criteria that distinguish 'normal' from 'abnormal'; that through diagnosis the condition should be defined; that rules governing treatment and management should be identified, and that these rules 'prescribed' by the physician should be followed. In some illnesses, however, medical criteria for defining the 'disorder' and providing a framework of knowledge with which it (and its social consequences) can be understood are a great deal more problematic.

One such case is epilepsy in children where the doctor often cannot, and 'will not', provide information about the nature of the disorder and its implications that would enable a family to make sense of, cope with and organise their social activities accordingly. Under such conditions, although the physician's claim to competence  may initially be taken for granted, his performance is ultimately critically appraised, his significance decreases, and alternative sources of knowledge are consulted, a process that is both a consequence of the doctor's 'failure' to provide information and a source of increasing challenge to, and contradiction of, the medical definition.

I do not wish to suggest that this always occurs, but that it does so in one form or another with considerable regularity. To illustrate this process, some examples of doctor—parent encounters will be presented, from a total of sixty-four documented observations. These depict stages in the child's 'career' as patient from the first time he attends out-patients clinics, through routine follow-up visits, to discharge. The exchanges took place in the presence of the observer and were written down as far as was possible word for word. The analysis of the observational material has been particularly informed by Scheff's work on the negotiation of definitions of the situation by participants (Scheff, 1968), and by the distinction made between a 'presented' as opposed to a 'believed' definition of reality (Wellman, 1969).

In addition, there are twenty-four families (twenty-six children) constituting the major study group who were selected as they attended the same hospital. The children are almost all in the age range eleven to nineteen and all have a 'primary' diagnosis of epilepsy. At least one member of the family (usually the mother) has been interviewed at home on one or more occasions, using a semi-structured approach. These interviews were taped and some aspects of parental accounts of contact with the medical profession are reported here.

THE MEDICAL CONSTRUCTION OF EPILEPSY — THE PROBLEM OF UNCERTAINTY

Before looking at interactions between doctors and parents, it is important to indicate briefly some of the problems doctors face in constructing and communicating a definition of the situation.

The concept of epilepsy held by the medical profession is a very good example of the way only certain phenomena from a potentially much wider range come to be identified and defined in diagnosis. While five to seven per cent of children are estimated to have seizures between birth and five years (*British Medical Journal*, 1972), not all are diagnosed as having epilepsy. For example, a clinical category, 'febrile convulsions', which is usually presumed to have a relatively benign outcome (though this is debated within the profession: see Millichap, 1968), identifies children whose seizures occur with high temperature. The medical criteria distinguishing epilepsy from febrile convulsions are, however, frankly problematic and also reflect the physician's awareness of the social implications of the term 'epilepsy'.

Most of the doctors in the hospital where the present study took place adopt a similar kind of working rule, which occurs in the context of what will be termed a strategy of 'normalisation'.

Not only is there an absence of consensus as to what epilepsy is and is not, but there is genuine uncertainty in making decisions about the precise nature of the seizures, and in predicting whether or not seizures will recur. Thus, although certain rules of thumb may be used, based on the results of medical research and the physician's own experience, it is often extremely difficult to make predictions about individual cases. There are also problems of diagnosis, and doctors may try to avoid naming the disorder because of the meaning it apparently conveys to parents.

Against the background of clinical uncertainty, the physician's claim to competence appears more problematic than in cases where he can be more 'successful'. Under such conditions, we might therefore expect his professional authority to be open to question, and that in encounters with parents he would tend to resort to strategies that as far as possible preserve the legitimacy of his position. The situation has evident parallels to the study conducted by Davis (1960).

With this in mind, we should assess what actually happens when the doctor and the parents of an epileptic child interact, and see to what extent the former is successful in preserving his claim to competence. We should also remember the problems the doctor faces when considering parental accounts of his performance.

## INITIAL CONTACT

Although for almost all parents a seizure is a frightening experience, often raising the idea that their child is dying or likely to suffer some permanent damage, the variability of the form it can take means that it is not always identified as 'epileptic'. One of the reasons for this is the commonly held stereotype that epileptic fits involve gross body movement, falling down, frothing at the mouth and so on. The existence of such a powerful stereotype, and parents' 'appeal' to it to provide an alternative definition to epilepsy, is in itself a potential source of conflict with the doctor. However, even where the event itself is evidently convulsive, it still does not mean that parents hold an initial definition of 'epilepsy' since the meaning this conveys is often quite different from other terms such as 'convulsions'.

All but two of the twenty-six children in the major group were referred to hospital by the family practitioner, the majority shortly after the initial episode. The other two were admitted to hospital directly. Little is known about the nature of the interaction between parents and general practitioner (GP), but parents claim that he plays a very marginal part both in respect of offering a diagnosis and in providing a set of rules for coping with the problems. It appears that, as the referral agent, the GP essentially transfers responsibility for these matters to the hospital.

The first attendance at hospital is therefore crucial for the parents since they expect the doctor to provide an explanation for the event, and to define what it signifies for the child and family. With few exceptions, it is the longest lasting encounter, generally taking between thirty and forty minutes, whereas routine follow-up appointments may not exceed five minutes. It is usually the only occasion a patient is guaranteed access to the consultant paediatrician, thereafter seeing a variety of different doctors (Ross, 1974; HMSO, 1969).

Typically, the initial encounter is highly structured and can be divided into a number of stages — the history-taking (usually recorded by a clinical assistant or a student); an examination performed by the assistant; the transfer to the consultant who will check details of the 'history'; a second examination; and finally a 'prescriptive' episode in which a 'diagnosis' is offered and rules of treatment and management identified.

In a sense, the history-taking sets a precedent for what follows, because almost immediately the doctor proceeds with questions about birth and development, diseases, immunisations and so on. This is the kind of interaction described by Coulthard and Ashby in this volume, a sequence of 'transfer' and 'matching' exchanges which makes it extremely difficult for parents to initiate anything other than 'complementary' definitions of the situation. The pattern is similar when questioning turns to the immediate problem, but an interesting process unfolds concerning the precise definition of the seizure event. Doctors tend to use words like 'turns', 'attacks' and, less frequently, 'convulsions', terms that do not presuppose a specific diagnostic category, and carry a more neutral connotation. It is as if they were 'feeling' for the parents' own definition, and once established utilise it in the ensuing course of the interaction. Almost always it is the parent who provides the definition which the doctor will then follow. In many respects the process has similarities with that described by Balint (1957) as a negotiation of illness until each participant agrees on a definition, but it also provides the doctor with an opportunity to avoid a specific commitment to the epilepsy diagnosis, and is part of a general orientation of 'normalisation'.

The use of such non-emotive terms throughout the interview is related to the conclusions drawn by the doctor as he turns from the examination to the 'prescriptive' phase. Usually the 'diagnosis' constitutes a summary of previously negotiated terms and is in effect a 'quasi-diagnosis' because it is always conditional on the results of the electroencephalogram (EEG) and of the skull X-ray, which are routine procedures used to supplement diagnostic decisions. It is a provisional definition which is potentially open to re-negotiation when additional information has become available. It has parallels with Bloor's analysis (in this volume) of the way 'disposal decisions' about tonsillectomy are delayed until the results of certain investigations are known.

Following the 'quasi-diagnosis', the doctor then moves to the area of prescription. Parents are usually told that their child should take 'routine medicine' for a minimum period of two years (irrespective of the results of the EEG). They are rarely informed of possible side effects. In addition, the doctor also specifies whether or not the child should be restricted in his activities. This is sometimes open to negotiation, as the following example illustrates.

*Doctor:* And I don't think you need restrict his activities at all really.

*Father:* Right.

*Doctor:* And they occur at night. If they do tend to recur, we may have to think again.

*Father:* Oh I'm not too worried about it.

*Doctor:* Mm. And if he goes swimming?

*Father:* He goes swimming. It's very well supervised. I don't think that there's much of a problem there.

*Doctor:* Good. OK. Any problems?

*Father:* No. I'm happy with the way things have gone.

In this case the father successfully negotiates an outcome which is substantiated by the doctor. In others, there is more of an 'ought' attached to the doctor's decision, but in no instance have parents been observed to question directly either the medication rule or any rules governing exclusion of the child from 'normal' activities.

The manner in which the doctor communicates such rules is often indecisive, almost apologetic. In addition, throughout the prescriptive phase of the interview the doctor emphasises that the child should continue to be treated as normal.

Finally, in respect of prognosis, it seems likely that the doctor's routine use of the medication rule (two years free of seizures) serves to indicate by implication that the 'disorder' may persist. However, with the general exception of younger children who have had 'febrile convulsions', about which doctors are more confident in their predictions, no more explicit guarantee is given since doctors are genuinely uncertain. To volunteer a more specific prognosis at this stage would risk a charge of lack of competence should they be proved wrong. The 'procrastination' of prognostic statements therefore is a means by which doctors preserve their 'functional autonomy'. It seems probable that the avoidance of the term 'epilepsy' ('a long-term thing') and the emphasis on 'normalisation' tend to generate a parental definition approximating to the 'normal' convulsion with the connotation of a relatively 'good' prognosis.

To sum up, the first interview, which is a crucial definitional encounter for the parents, is characterised by a rigid structure where parents have only a limited opportunity to initiate anything other than complementary definitions. They *appear* remarkably passive in this interview. The physician's tight control on the proceedings does not imply however that parents are provided with specific information about the diagnosis or a more general framework of knowledge for understanding and coping with epilepsy. The doctor avoids committing himself to a specific diagnosis, and the summary is clearly provisional in that it depends on the results of tests, and is thus potentially open to re-negotiation on a subsequent occasion. Similarly, except for the medication rule, which implicitly provides some prognostic guidelines, the doctor avoids any specific commitment to prediction of the outcome. Rules governing medication and the social activities of the child are provided by the doctor, sometimes appearing open to negotiation, and are communicated in the context of a general process of normalisation.

## LATER CONTACTS

Following the EEG, patients begin what is often a succession of visits. If the EEG result has proved to be satisfactory, this is often emphasised to support a normalisation process, but this does not mean that the medical diagnosis of epilepsy is negated or that the child is not prescribed medication. 'Abnormal' results are communicated in a style that plays down the significance of the term, as it might be used to make further evaluations of the child. For instance:

*Doctor:*    She had this brain-wave test as you know, and there were some abnormalities that showed up — that goes hand in hand with a fit — but it's nothing to worry about.

Generally speaking, doctors still tend to maintain tight control over the encounter, but the following example illustrates that even in the initial stages of a patient's career parents do take the initiative and are not deterred by 'inhibitory routines'. In this case, concerning a ten-year-old boy who had been admitted following a convulsion, the mother is very insistent, 'forcing' answers from the doctor who is unable to prevent her sustaining the challenge. The outcome essentially reasserts the *status quo*, but she is at least partially successful in obtaining a diagnosis however implicitly it is conveyed.

*Doctor:*    [looking at the notes in front of him] — And he's only ever had this one convulsion.

*Mother:*    Well two actually.

*Doctor:*    Well his EEG is within normal limits for his age.

*Mother:*    Well what's *that* supposed to mean?

*Doctor:*    Well — it's a bit like the electrocardiogram, you know, when they take an electrical reading from the heart and they can see whether there is an abnormality. In some children with epilepsy and convulsions it can show if there's a small part of the brain which acts as a kind of trigger.

*Mother:*    But we don't know whether or not it is a convulsion. We want to know if it's epilepsy or a convulsion. So, we're very up in the air I'm afraid.

*Doctor:*    I know, I know — obviously what we need is a good eye-witness.

*Mother:*    That's right. It's only fortunate that his brother sleeps in the same room.

*Doctor:*    Well. Convulsions are shaking — epilepsy can include convulsions but it can apply to other kinds of phenomena, to other kinds of things [pauses]. Epilepsy has this aura about it, they talk about it in hushed terms don't they?

*Mother:*    Yes, they do.

*Doctor:*    It's like TB used to be years ago, isn't it? But where does this get us?

*Mother:*    Well exactly, but — we want to know. His teacher wants to know if he can go swimming. We've told his teacher, I must say I don't like the idea of his being on tablets for the rest of his life.

*Doctor:*    No I know — [to the boy]: Let's have a look at you shall we Peter? [he proceeds with a brief examination].

Some parents remain very passive in encounters with doctors even when they have been attending the out-patient clinic for quite some time, but open bargaining can occur, making this a major, if not the most usual, development. This is particularly apparent when the doctor fails to control the seizures, or when he recommends some major reorganisation of a child's life such as transfer to special school or admission of the child for investigation of poor seizure control.

For instance, many parents claim that the drugs their child is on have quite marked side effects, added to which is the symbolic significance attributed to 'being on tablets'. They may therefore attempt to challenge the doctor in respect of the medication rule. Generally they are unsuccessful, but sometimes obtain a compromise, as in the following example:

*Doctor:* There've been no further episodes since she's been taking the medicine.

*Mother:* No, it's all been quite successful. Do you think it would be possible to reduce the dosage? She's not had any . . . .

*Doctor:* Well she's on a very low dose anyway. If anything it's too low for *petit mal.*

*Mother:* Well would it be possible to have tablets instead of medicine? The medicine's so sticky. They must put masses of sugar in it.

*Doctor:* Yes I don't see why not. I think we can arrange that — [then addressing the girl]: what would *you* prefer Sarah, tablets or medicine?

*Patient:* [hesitates and looks at mother] Tablets.

*Mother:* How do we know if she's still having them? I mean if she's still on drugs? Is there a period of time? I mean if the *petit mal* is over, we won't know, will we? The drugs don't really cure her, they just stop it showing, and we couldn't know that if she was still on them. . . . .

*Doctor:* Well no, it's not quite like that. She should remain on drugs for at least six months, more likely one year. We'll repeat the EEG then and see what's what. You see, something definitely showed up and usually there's no change — the EEG's not a very useful test, but it's a pointer . . . [pause]. I'll tell you what we'll do, we'll compromise. We'll make it nine months. . . .

At this consultation the doctor uses his knowledge about drug dosage to overcome the mother's definition. She does however obtain some changes (though it is interesting to speculate what the outcome would have been had the child not answered as she did), and after a highly pertinent question about the persistence of the underlying condition, she obtains an account (explanation) from the doctor which reinforces the modified medication rule. The doctor offers a compromise which goes some way towards meeting her case.

Occasionally, parents offer a definition that effects a major change in the doctor's policy. One such instance concerns a nine-year-old boy who had been diagnosed epileptic since he was very young, though the type of seizure was atypical and had proved an intractable medical problem. He was accompanied by both parents and observed at the twenty-first consultation. An exceptional continuity of treatment had been maintained, and he had seen only three doctors, largely because one of them had become especially interested in him. On this occasion, the doctor makes a remarkable admission.

The relationship between the doctor and parents is extremely informal by comparison with most others, and the first part of the interview is taken up with an exchange of jokes and pleasantries. Then, the doctor initiates a loosely structured exchange about recent seizure history which brings forth the response that the last 'major' attack occurred four months previously.

*Father:*    He did have one which was different. He seemed to lose his balance, be unsteady on his feet and just fall over . . . [pause]. I thought the drugs had no side effects.
*Doctor:*    Which drugs?
*Father:*    Epanutin.
*Doctor:*    Oh, all drugs have side effects.

The exchange then turns to a consideration of how the child is developing, the parents offering an account that stresses considerable improvement.

*Doctor:*    Well, I'm rather impressed with how he's getting on. I think we'll take him off Epanutin. Indeed, perhaps off all drugs. How do you feel about that?
*Mother:*    We're willing to try.
*Father:*    We've never been very convinced that it has any effect anyway.
*Doctor:*    Well, nor am I. Now let's see if we take him off . . . .

After the doctor has specified exactly how the drugs will be reduced, the mother again reinforces the parental (and by now mutual) definition that the child is improving. The doctor again substantiates this in no uncertain manner.

Doctor:    I've seen some remarkable recoveries when children are taken off drugs. I think he's doing very well. All right then, we'll see you in two months shall we and see how things are going.

This is not only an interesting, if unusual, example of successful negotiation on the part of parents, but the 'admission' by the doctor that the very treatment for epilepsy might have disadvantages that outweigh the benefits stands in stark contrast to the exchanges that occur when children first attend hospital. The medication rule is defined quite routinely; there is little or no discussion of possible side effects, and almost always parents are not offered a choice as to whether the child should receive medication. It is only as parents become more experienced in coping with and evaluating their child's epilepsy that they begin to initiate challenges to the doctor. Simultaneously, it becomes increasingly difficult for the doctor to utilise a highly structured interview to inhibit the emergence of parental definitions. He is 'forced' to open up the agenda, to provide information which hitherto had not been offered. It is no longer possible for him to take for granted that his competence is assumed — he must 'work' for it.

Consider the following instance where a fifteen-year-old girl with 'chronic' epilepsy who has attended out-patients on numerous occasions over a period of four years, and has been admitted several times, confronts the doctor over the question of whether or not they will ever find a solution to her problem.

Patient:    Will they ever go?
Doctor:    Yes they will. We'll get them under control. There are so many different types of drugs and it's a matter of finding the right one. We'll find the right one, don't worry.
Mother:    The one she had this morning was, well, terrible, frightening really. She was out and thrashing about. She didn't know what was happening.
Doctor:    OK, Mary. We *will* get them under control. We will. *What is so important is to have confidence in us and yourself.* . . .

In this case, the doctor is 'obliged' to construct his claim to expertise and to spell out one of the features of the doctor—patient relationship that is understood to be crucial, namely that patients must have confidence in the physician. As far as the ensuing exchange is concerned, neither the mother nor the patient further question his competence, and to that extent the doctor is (formally) successful.

However, the following example illustrates that parents may remain unconvinced, and 'force' the doctor to recognise the validity of their own definitions. This interaction between a doctor and mother concerns an eleven-year-old boy who was attending out-patients for the thirty-fourth time in four years. He has continued to have seizures despite various doctors' attempts to find an effective drug, virtually all anticonvulsants having been tried unsuccessfully. The boy has also for some time been recommended for transfer to a special school, a decision resisted by the mother.

Early on in the encounter, the mother lets the doctor know that she possesses a substantial knowledge about epilepsy (she knows the medical terms), and volunteers her own definition as to why there has been some recent improvement ('going to the toilet regularly'), a definition that is accepted by the doctor. The latter, however, strongly suggests that an improvement in seizure control is essential and offers a list of available drugs that the mother could choose from. The boy has been on them all.

| | |
|---|---|
| *Doctor:* | We must stop them altogether. |
| *Mother:* | Oh you'll never stop them. They've tried everything. It's no good drugging him up to the eyeballs. He's going through a bad patch now but he has good times as well. |
| *Doctor:* | What do you do when he has the bad patches? |
| *Mother:* | I just keep him home for a while. |
| *Doctor:* | How is his schooling? |
| *Mother:* | All right. He can read. His mentality is good, you can see that — it's just the drugs. |
| *Doctor:* | [to the patient] Can you write a story for me — about the hospital perhaps? [The boy grins but does not respond. Then, turning back to mother]. It is obviously in a way unsatisfactory to see a new doctor. |
| *Mother:* | I don't mind going over the details again. |
| *Doctor:* | [emphatically] We've got to make a big effort to stop the attacks. |

*Mother:*  You can try. I'm willing to give it a go.

*Doctor:*  What do the school say?

*Mother:*  They want him to go to a school for epileptics — I'm *not* going to allow it. I've got all his papers and everything through [for normal secondary school]. There's other children up there with epilepsy. No problem! Anyway half the kids who go there can't read or write. I think I've got a good case. I know he'd get more individual attention but I'm willing to take a risk. I know he'll get lost there but. . . .

The doctor intervenes and does not attempt to argue against the mother's definition of the situation. Instead, he takes a blood sample, and returns to the issue of changing to another drug.

*Mother:*  Oh no — they did this when he was in hospital. It was cruel, it really was. They chopped and changed all the time. Look at him now, he's all drugged up.
[The doctor then gets the patient to walk along a straight line, checking for side effects. He is noticeably unsteady and attempts to maintain his balance by clutching onto the wall.]

*Doctor:*  Does he go through phases of being unsteady like this?

*Mother:*  He's like that all the time.

*Doctor:*  It may be that during the summer holiday . . . .

*Mother:*  Never. Never.

*Doctor:*  But we've got to control them.

*Mother:*  No. No. He always comes out worse than he went in.

*Doctor:*  Well OK. But we must try and cut them down when he goes to the new school.

*Mother:*  Really, bringing him in is an absolute waste of time.

The doctor does not pursue the argument any further. He simply asks her if she needs a further supply of tablets and suggests that the patient returns in two months time. Ironically, the mother requests that the appointment be fixed for four rather than eight weeks. As mother and patient leave, the doctor raises his eyes in a gesture of despair.

This is rather an extreme example but it does indicate the pattern that can develop between doctor and parent, particularly when the child continues to have seizures and some major issue such as social relocation occurs. Not only do we see the parent initiating questions and challenges which may or may not be successfully negotiated, but the doctor cannot rely solely on routine solutions to substantiate the medical definition of the situation. He has to 'work' increasingly to maintain his claim to competence. What occurs over time is a gradual release of information about diagnosis, prognosis, treatment and management, information that is initially not provided. Usually it is the parent rather than the doctor who effects this communication. While it is true that the clinical uncertainty doctors face is a real problem, the strategies adopted to overcome this (not 'telling', normalisation etc.) actually create and perpetuate the uncertainty parents experience. Once information is released, it places the doctor in a kind of 'double-bind' situation, because parents think the doctor has hitherto concealed the knowledge they require. This increases the parents' bargaining position on subsequent occasions, particularly when they encounter a new doctor who may attempt to rely on routine solutions.

The position of the doctor *vis-à-vis* parents may change, sometimes quite dramatically. Even when parents remain apparently passive, we should not assume that they are not assessing the situation critically. They may 'present' a definition in the context of the doctor—patient interview to which they are not committed 'outside the clinic'.

## PARENTAL ACCOUNTS OF DOCTOR'S PERFORMANCE

Webb and Stimson have argued (in this volume) that people's accounts of consultations with doctors stand in contrast to observations of what happens. In the account, patients are depicted as much more active than they actually are and doctors are described in essentially derogatory terms which detract from their formal public image. These authors believe that the story is a vehicle for expressing sentiments not manifest in the encounter itself, and for redressing the apparent inequality between doctor and patient.

Accounts given by parents of an epileptic child have similarities with those described by these authors. In the present case, however, the nature of the relationship between doctor and parent often *does* change over time and *is* different from the single consultation with the general practitioner. I suggest that the stories given by these parents are not merely constructed for the benefit of the interviewer (though this is an important consideration), but represent a process of assessment of and reflection about their own position as parents attempting to cope with the child, and the corresponding performance of the physician as 'expert'. It is not only that the accounts constitute statements that bridge the gap between action and expectation (Scott and Lyman, 1968), but that as an evaluation of preceding interactions they provide a basis for future action *in* the situation of encounter with the doctor. Or, rather than effecting a change in their future presentations to the doctor, they may sustain a definition of the situation corresponding to that held by the doctor, while 'believing' in another, and acting according to the 'privately' held definition.

Most parents claim that the diagnosis of epilepsy was given by the doctor only because they 'forced' it from him, or that it was released by one or other doctor when the child had already been attending for quite a long time. They often express the view that the diagnosis must have been known, a position that contrasts with that of the doctor who may have been uncertain about the nature of the disorder and clinical prognosis. For instance:

*Mother:* . . . and I think it was only about 2 visits ago that one of the doctors said to me 'Did I know what was supposed to be wrong with her' and actually I thought I knew because a friend of mine had told me that this is what it sounded like, a very mild epilepsy, and it wasn't until then that this doctor said 'Do you know what's supposed to be wrong with her'. I don't think up until then that anybody had mentioned that she was supposed to have had a mild epilepsy.

Another example illustrates the problem parents face when the terms used by doctors actually perpetuate uncertainty. A nineteen-year-old girl had been having what her mother described as 'fainting fits' from seven years of age. Finally, when she had an attack in public, they felt the time had come to find out exactly what the disorder was. The parents claim they received differing and evasive accounts from the GP, school medical officer and hospital. In respect of the former,

*Father:* I'm a bit biased. I think doctors should tell you, but I don't think you should have to ask them. Of course you

Father:   can't go by our doctor 'cos he doesn't tell you anything anyway.

Mother:   No, but I had to ask him.

Father:   I had to literally browbeat him. He's getting on, he's a fusser. I asked him 'for goodness sake doctor, calm down', I said. 'You're making me bloody nervous,' I said. 'I want to speak to you', I said. 'Sit down quiet while I speak, will you'. He sat down then.

Mother:   When he told me she was epileptic, I said I wouldn't go out of the surgery until he told me. I said 'I want to know. I got a right to know.'

Author:   What particularly did you want to know then?

Mother:   Well if she was definitely epileptic, because of the school, you see, they were pressuring us about her going to college.

It is not only the issue of diagnosis that constitutes a problem for both parties; parents look to the doctor to provide a framework of knowledge around which they can understand epilepsy and learn to cope with it. Often they perceive that such information is either not being volunteered or that when challenged doctors appear evasive.

Such overtly critical attitudes lead parents to initiate challenges to the doctor, opening up the agenda and creating the situation where the doctor has to 'work' to construct his claim to competence. Many perceive, at least implicitly, the doctor attempting to maintain his professional status, but none put it as well as the following parents, who incidentally claim the treatment they have received could not have been better.

Father:   Well, I mean, quite honestly I think often the reason doctors don't reveal, or reveal a minimum, is that they don't want to face all the follow-up questions which will arise out of this. It's not just a matter of time, it's just that if you're explaining something, it's got to be — I mean, you're a professional man and you — if you explain in detail you're almost revealing the secrets of your profession.

Why do these 'dissatisfied' parents continue to attend hospital out-patients? First, it seems that once the relationship has been entered into there is a kind of obligation on the part of parents to continue to maintain it, although not in the sense of the 'sick-role' formulation (Parsons, 1951). It is more critically evaluated than that implies. Second, some parents hold the definition that, unless they are seen to preserve attachment to the doctor, they may forgo the right to have medical treatment at all; the doctor's 'ultimate weapon'. Third is the attitude that, although at present doctors may not be in a position to provide a solution to the child's problem, this might be remedied.

In a situation of uncertainty parents turn to alternative sources of knowledge (e.g. lay networks) in the attempt to obtain answers they appear not to be getting from doctors. In part, this process reflects the increasingly marginal significance of the physician, at the same time providing a means by which medical definitions can be assessed. Occasionally, an alternative definition of the disorder emerges and is sustained by an 'appeal' to the stereotype (conflicting with the typical fit), but there are other areas that indicate the absence of commitment to rules provided by the doctor, notably rules governing the taking of medication and those concerned with the child's participation in certain social activities.

With regard to the former, it is assumed from the doctor's point of view that those parents who fail to administer the drugs are in some way 'bad' or 'inadequate', but considered against the background of interaction with and assessment of the physician the picture can look rather different (Stimson, 1974). Most parents admit that occasionally the child has failed to take the prescribed medication either because they 'forgot' or because the child developed some particular strategy for avoiding ingestion. There are however a number of instances where a more conscious decision was made to contravene the medication rule; a decision that constitutes a definition of the situation in conflict with that held by the medical profession. Interestingly, in these cases the 'break' is not total.

A fourteen-year-old girl had been having seizures on and off since she was three, and lately with considerable frequency. Initially, her mother took no action because two other children had similar episodes and 'grew out of them'. Following a severe attack for which she was hospitalised, epilepsy was diagnosed and appropriate medication prescribed. Soon afterwards, her mother took her off tablets because there were no symptoms. The girl took no medication for five years, during which time she apparently had no further seizures, *but*, in order to maintain the appearance of the 'good' mother, she regularly went to her GP to obtain repeat prescriptions.

What she was doing in effect was presenting a definition of the situation that accorded with that of the doctor while privately 'believing' another. Latterly, because of recurrence, the girl takes medication but other rules governing participation in social activities are ignored.

It is not my intention to suggest that the contravention of medical rules always occurs, but it does illustrate that the significance of the physician as rule-provider is subject to limitations. It indicates that parents do not simply take for granted the right of doctors to define the disorder and provide prescriptions for action. They utilise their own experience of 'the child having a seizure', their knowledge of epilepsy derived from sources other than the medical profession, and their assessment of the doctor's performance to construct definitions of the situation. It is a much more dynamic process than that provided by the 'sick-role' construct.

CONCLUSION

This chapter provides some observations about the significance of the physician in constructing a definition of the situation for parents of an epileptic child. Usually, in medical sociology the physician's role is accorded considerable significance, and he is understood to create by his diagnosis a particular social status for the patient, with implications for his everyday life. Such a theoretical framework assumes either a remarkably normative orientation (as in Parsons' work), or implicitly, that the physician is empowered to construct definitions that are usually taken for granted by the patient, or in this case his parents (Freidson, 1970). In either case the emphasis is overtly mechanistic. We do not see people thinking, reflecting, making sense of, working or negotiating in the context of their interations with the 'professional'. Neither do we see the doctor having to cope with clinical uncertainty and the interrelated problem of maintaining the legitimacy of his position as 'expert'. It is ultimately a process whereby parents may 'suspend belief' (Wagner, 1970) in the physician's competence, although preserving an attachment to official sources of knowledge.

Whether this is something that is peculiar to a condition where doctors face uncertainty, and is socially stigmatised, is an open question. It seems more likely that epilepsy is an archetype of the problematic construction and maintenance of medical definitions and solutions, a situation that may be paralleled in other professional—client encounters. It suggests that we should direct our attention towards the way in which the definitions offered by professionals are created, and under what conditions they are sustained.

## NOTES

1 This study was originally funded by the Epilepsy Research Fund of the British Epilepsy Association, and is now supported by the Social Science Research Council.

# 3 School Placement: Interactions Between Doctors and Mothers of Physically Handicapped Children

## by Elizabeth M. Anderson

### INTRODUCTION

This chapter is about the nature of communications between doctors and mothers of physically handicapped children of normal or borderline normal intelligence at the crucial point at which a decision about school placement has to be made. Usually school medical officers or medical officers of health (now called community physicians) are most involved, although hospital consultants and general practitioners may also offer or be called upon for advice. At this time (as at many other points in the life of a congenitally physically handicapped child) the doctors are part of the rehabilitative rather than the curative medical services, the aim of such services being 'to gradually increase the level of behavioural functioning, or to provide compensation for the handicap where possible' and to 'help handicapped people to achieve a maximum degree of independence and acceptance' (Kennedy, 1973).

### SCHOOL PLACEMENT PROCEDURES: THEORY AND PRACTICE

Although most of this chapter is about factors that influence mother—doctor communications regarding school placement, it is important first of all to be clear about how the placement works in theory and in practice. In theory, placement should result from a team decision to which parents, doctors, psychologists, teachers, social workers and administrators all contribute. Discussions should begin early on, and the child's educational needs should be stressed.

In practice, findings in my own study of disabled children (Anderson, 1973) and in Sheila Hewett's (1970) study of cerebral-palsied children indicated that discussions about school placement were often not initiated until the child was well into his fourth year or even later. The final decision often appeared to rest upon one examination by a local authority medical officer of health, made during a brief visit to the child's home or in a clinic, although psychologists or hospital consultants might also be involved. The purpose of the visit to the home is often merely to complete the statutory forms and to underwrite a prior decision. As a result, parents naturally tend to feel that the decision is a sudden one and that their point of view has not been fully considered. Full consultation between all those with useful knowledge about the child is rare, and school heads are much more likely to be informed rather than consulted about the placement of a child in their school.

Local authorities vary enormously, and in many instances placement procedures may approximate much more closely to the ideal set out in the Younghusband report (1970). This should be improved following the Department of Education and Science (1975) circular stressing the contribution parents, psychologists and teachers, as well as doctors, have to make to assessment procedures. Even so, decisions about placement made by doctors still, in fact, carry enormous weight. The practitioner—parent relationship and the nature of the communications between them about placement are therefore of great importance.

RESEARCH ON PARENTAL ATTITUDES

Although the literature on the social, emotional and educational adjustment of physically handicapped children is extensive (see Pilling's annotated bibliographies, 1972, 1973a, 1973b), little research has been done on how mothers perceive the process of rearing a physically handicapped child.

My own study (Anderson, 1973) of the integration of physically handicapped children included interviews with ninety-nine mothers of disabled children aged five to ten years old who had ultimately been placed in ordinary primary schools. Most of the children were of normal intelligence although some were of 'borderline-ESN' ability. The most frequent handicaps were congenital abnormalities (30 per cent), cerebral palsy (22 per cent) and spina bifida (16 per cent). Seventeen per cent of the children were mildly, 61 per cent moderately and 22 per cent severely handicapped.

Although the main emphasis in the study was on the school attainments and social adjustment of the children and on the practical arrangements needed, the interview with the mother included a discussion of the child's school placement history, additional data being obtained from the children's records. Special school placement had been suggested for over half of the sample by a variety of professional health workers. The strength of the recommendation and the persistence parents displayed in order to obtain ordinary school placement varied greatly. Case history material was collected on the practical problems they had encountered and their attitudes towards special school placement were explored. Overall, only 5 per cent favoured special school placement, with 15 per cent uncommitted and 80 per cent opposed.

PARENT—DOCTOR COMMUNICATIONS ABOUT SCHOOL PLACEMENT

When a mother and doctor meet to resolve a problem concerning a handicapped child, what sort of factors are likely to affect the nature and quality of their interaction? The specific situation discussed here is the visit of a local authority medical officer to the mother at home to obtain information to make a decision (either by himself alone, or with the mother or other professionals) about the most appropriate school placement for the child. The mother—doctor interaction is only part of the placement procedure, but usually a very central part. Although what is said here refers in particular to physically handicapped children who are 'marginal' in terms of the likelihood of their being placed in an ordinary or in a special school, much of it is applicable to children handicapped in other ways.

Below are set out in diagrammatic form the main stages in the mother—doctor meeting. (Tait, 1973, has proposed something rather similar for what he describes as the 'behavioural aspects' of patient—doctor consultations.) The two main participants need not of course always be the mother and the doctor. Fathers, and the children themselves, have major roles to play. Similarly, the doctor has been selected as the other main participant, although much of what follows is applicable to the mother's interaction with other professionals, particularly psychologists.

In Figure 1 the mother—doctor consultation is shown as falling into three main stages. While this is obviously a simplification, since there is much blurring between them, it provides a useful way of analysing what is happening.

Stage A represents the point at which the participants meet, often, in this situation, for the first (and only) time. This is the most crucial stage, since unless a satisfactory relationship is formed it is unlikely that either of the participants will be able to gather information that will enable them to come to a mutually satisfactory solution. Unfortunately, as indicated in Figure 1 and discussed in more detail below, this stage may be omitted. Preconceptions of each participant about the other, lack of training in interpersonal skills on the doctor's part, pressure of time or even the fact that the real purpose of the meeting is simply to ratify a decision that has already been

*Figure 1*     *Stages in the mother—doctor interaction*

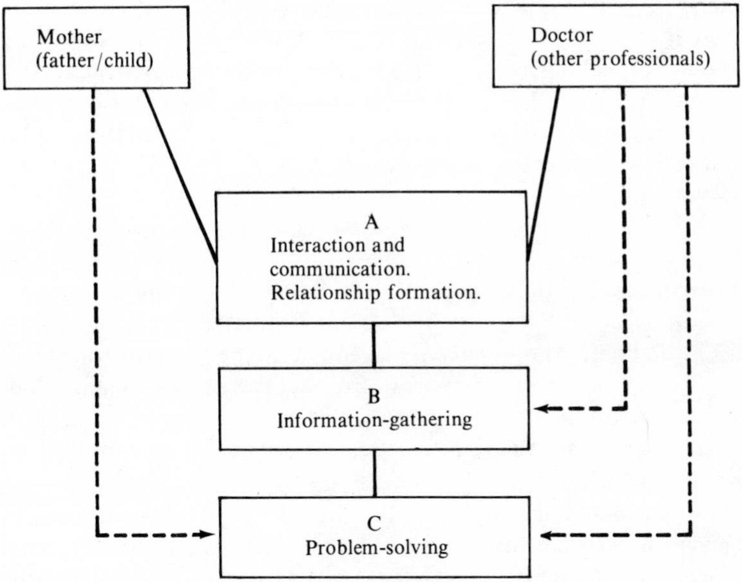

taken may mean that the participants proceed to stage B or even to C without any understanding of the needs and expectations of the other.

At stage B both participants are attempting to gather information. However, as Dembo (1964) puts it, doctors believe 'the purpose of the meeting to be a systematic and rational evaluation of factual information. The parent, while agreeing with this aim, has another goal in mind; support for the view that the child is not as handicapped as he appears, that something can be done to help the handicap and that the professional can point to ways to provide that help.' In particular, in the situation under discussion here, the mother wants information about the different types of schooling available.

Participants come to a decision regarding school placement at stage C. Ideally, there is mutual agreement, or a decision may be postponed until further information has been gathered. Unfortunately, two other outcomes are also common. First, a decision may be taken, but one of the participants — more often the mother — feels pressurised into accepting an unwanted 'solution'. Second, no decision may be taken with the conflict between the doctor's recommendation and the mother's wishes openly expressed. In such situations mothers may be labelled as 'irrational' or 'unrealistic' while doctors may be accused of 'not wanting to know', of making major decisions on the basis of one fleeting visit, of underestimating the child's assets and overestimating his liabilities, of using 'unfair' tests, of giving conflicting advice or of treating the mother in a generally unsympathetic way.

MOTHER—DOCTOR CONFLICTS OVER SCHOOL PLACEMENT

Why do conflicts over school placement (in the form of either overt clashes or hidden resentment) so frequently arise? Two major kinds of 'explanation' can be given. The first is in terms of gaps or inadequacies in the existing services available to mothers of handicapped children.

In my own interviews with mothers the most frequently voiced problems were lack of advice on school placement, lateness of advice (near child's fifth birthday), contradictory advice (from professionals), failure of professionals to consult parents fully about their wishes, the need for parents to 'put up a fight' to override the recommendation for special school placement, and practical difficulties in arranging ordinary school placement even when the mother and doctor agree that this is appropriate.

The second kind of 'explanation' of mother—doctor conflicts over school placement and the one looked at more closely in this chapter focuses on the mother—doctor interaction itself, and on the way in which the different needs and expectations of the participants impede satisfactory relationship formation and minimise rather than optimise the amount of relevant information that is gathered. Several major factors have been selected which may have a harmful effect on stage A, stage B and both stages A and B of the interaction. These are not discussed in order of importance, since this is likely to vary with the individuals concerned, and with the nature and severity of the child's disability; nor is the list intended to be an exhaustive one, the focus being more on the mother's rather than the doctor's perception of the situation.

## FACTORS AFFECTING STAGE A, RELATIONSHIP FORMATION

Three important factors affecting the behaviour of the participants are:

(i) the mother's prior experience of the medical profession and the extent to which she now perceives doctors and perhaps other professionals as supportive or hostile;
(ii) her perception of the school placement decision as a 'crisis' point in the child's history;
(iii) the doctor's perception of this particular mother and of how she fits into his concept of the 'good' mother.

### (i) The mother's prior experience of the medical profession, and her perception of doctors and other professionals

For many mothers of physically handicapped children, in particular those whose children have congenital abnormalities such as spina bifida, the mother's first close contact with a doctor is at the birth crisis. Roskies (1972) found that the way this was handled was one of 'confusion, contradiction and ambivalence', with doctors tending to concentrate either on the affective needs of the mother or on the possibilities of help for the children.

When a child is born with cerebral palsy, a diagnosis is often not made till much later. Ninety per cent of the mothers in Hewett's (1970) study felt that something was wrong before the child was diagnosed as spastic, and the majority (70 per cent) felt that they had a right to information about their children as soon as the doctors suspected that something was wrong. The fact that many mothers knew that doctors had withheld information may well affect their perception of them during later assessments. From the doctor's viewpoint, 'stalling' about a diagnosis, as Voysey (1972b) points out, both   protects him against future error and enables him to avoid provoking unmanageable emotional reactions.

After the child's birth, most parents are in regular contact with hospital consultants. In addition to hospital and clinic staff, mothers are also often in fairly close contact with a GP. In Hewett's study the mothers' comments on helpful and unhelpful GPs (56 per cent found their GP helpful, 44 per cent unhelpful) indicated that the relationship was influenced greatly by the doctor's ability to convey the idea that he was an ally, working with the parents, not against them.

Clearly, in the early years, parents of handicapped children need and expect advice and support of a 'social work' nature from the medical profession. Walker *et al.* (1971) found that the greatest need among mothers with spina bifida children was for counselling, not only immediately following the birth but 'over a long-term period', and thought that 'until comprehensive community care is fully established this counselling should be provided by the hospital and in the parents' own homes'. Often the nature of the 'support' that parents require from doctors is simply the reassurance that they, as parents, are doing all that can be done for the child.

Unfortunately, many mothers of physically handicapped children appear to look on doctors as 'opponents rather than allies, to be approached with a mixture of caution and militance rather than confidence' (Hewett, 1970). The feeling that they have to 'fight' for their children is frequently encountered, and it is not surprising that at periods of 'stress', such as at the school placement 'crisis', this feeling is intensified.

*(ii) The mother's perception of the school placement decision as a 'crisis' point in the child's history*

Roskies's (1972) intensive interviews with the mothers of the thalidomide children show that a mother may regard the birth and rearing of a handicapped child as a series of crises, varying in the amount of tension they produce. First comes the birth; the next 'crisis' occurs when the mother returns home and has to initiate the child into the 'normal' community, while later attendance at a rehabilitation institute or hospital may constitute further crises.

For some mothers, the period when the child is about three to four-and-a-half years old may be one of relatively low tension, with 'the potent factor maintaining the mother's sense of tension . . . their fear of the future . . . would [society's tolerance] endure during the tests of school entry, adolescence, vocational adjustment and marriage?' (Roskies, 1972). Next to interviews on the birth period, the most anxiety-provoking topic for mothers was discussion of their future plans and expectations. The mothers who felt the most stress were those whose children were 'marginal' in terms of acceptance in the normal community. Their handicaps were too severe to 'pass' unnoticed, but not gross enough for the mothers to have given up hope of acceptance. For these mothers, 'education assumed a unique importance, both because they considered it one of the crucial tests in determining the child's relative normality, and also because they viewed education as one of the major means of compensating for a serious deviance.'

Professionals often appear to be unaware of the stressfulness of this issue for mothers. They are not entirely to blame, since on their part mothers often try to conceal the strength of their feelings, the better to play the role of the 'good' mother which society demands of them (see iii below) like the mother who confessed how, after the doctor's visit, she 'dreaded the postman coming every day in case there was a letter to say he had to go to a special school . . . [though] I tried to keep the worry to myself'.

*(iii) The doctor's perception of a particular mother and of how she fits into his concept of the 'good' mother*

For many medical officers of health, visiting a home to discuss the question of school placement may be the first — and sometimes the only — direct contact with the family. However, even in such a case, information provided by social workers, health visitors, hospital consultants and others will probably mean that the doctor already has certain expectations both about the child's physical and mental abilities and about the mother. She may well have already been labelled by him as 'over-protective', 'difficult', 'hostile' or 'co-operative'.

In addition to bringing these particular preconceptions to the meeting, the doctor, like other professionals, may have a clear concept of a 'good' mother. Roskies (1972) found that in practice a 'good' mother was someone who was able to adjust to the existing social system. In Roskies's study this was the Rehabilitation Institute of Montreal, but it might equally well be the existing structure of special education in an area. To adjust satisfactorily a mother had first to perceive the child as sufficiently abnormal to require rehabilitation (here the parallel would be special schooling), but as sufficiently normal to be integrated into the family and community. Second, she had to be involved enough with the child to participate fully in the rehabilitation programme but detached enough to permit lengthy separations (special boarding school placement would make a similar demand); and finally she had to be sufficiently passive to accept a dependent status at the Rehabilitation Institute — i.e. in her relationship with the professionals managing her child — but sufficiently active to function independently as the mother of the child in the home and community.

In Hewett's (1970) words,

> . . . the parents, and later the child himself, must walk a tight-rope between acceptance of the fact that he is different from other children and insistence that he should be like them in as many ways as possible. If they emphasize his differences, continuously 'make allowances' for his disability and learn a habit of helping and shielding they may be labelled as 'over-protective'; if they minimize his handicap, treat him as an ordinary member of his family and speak with optimism of his mental attainment or physical prospects they may be judged to have failed to accept the situation.

It is small wonder that mothers may be unable to play such a complex and contradictory role; an awareness on the doctor's part of what mothers are being asked to do might lessen some of the potential conflicts.

## FACTORS AFFECTING STAGE B, INFORMATION GATHERING

At stage B each of the participants may require two main kinds of information. First, both need information about the child's present level of functioning, in particular, when ordinary school placement is in question, about his intellectual level; and their differing perceptions of this may be a major source of conflict. The mother's perception of her child's intelligence level may be determined to a considerable extent by her need to focus on what is 'normal'. The doctor, on the other hand, may see the purpose of his visit to be the 'systematic collection and rational evaluation of factual information', which he may not be willing to discuss in detail with the mother. These factors are discussed under (i) and (ii) below.

Secondly, in stage B, information about different types of schooling that may be appropriate is being sought. The mother is likely to opt for the alternative that she sees as offering the child the best means of 'compensating' for his disability. In many cases this will appear as the ordinary school. The doctor is also concerned with the 'compensatory' role of schooling, but his perception of the alternative available may differ from the mother's. These factors are discussed under (iii) and (iv) below.

### (i) The mother's perception of her child's intelligence level and her need to focus on what is 'normal' in the child

When a mother and a doctor meet to discuss school placement the mother brings to the situation certain perceptions about her child's mental ability. These perceptions are closely related to her need to avoid identification with the community of the mentally retarded. Many research studies suggest that there is a strong tendency among mothers of physically handicapped children to overestimate their children's abilities (Boles, 1959; Jensen and Kogan, 1962; Dembo,

1964; Barclay and Vaught, 1964; Keith and Markie, 1969; Roskies, 1972; Tew, 1973). The tendency to overestimate ability is not confined to parents of children with spina bifida or cerebral palsy. Roskies (1972) found in her interviews with the mothers of thalidomide children that, when looking ahead to plans for schooling, few mothers considered intellectual ability as a relevant problem despite the fact that several children had scored in the borderline or retarded range.

General explanations can be offered for this tendency as well as explanations specific to particular handicaps. An example of the latter is Tew's finding (1973) that the mothers most likely to overestimate the intelligence of spina bifida children were those whose children showed the 'cocktail-party syndrome'. This pattern of hyper-verbal behaviour is seen in about a third of all children with spina bifida or hydrocephalus. Their verbal ability is apparently superior, although the content of what the child says and his comprehension of language may be poor. Not only mothers but paediatricians, teachers and others may be misled by the child's verbal fluency.

Where there is a specific reason for the mother's overestimation of a child's ability it should be possible to warn both her and other professionals against using this as the only yardstick in assessing mental ability. However, more general factors affecting her perception of the child's ability may also be operating. The child's developmental progress may differ from that of other children and the mother may see him as slow to develop rather than as limited in ability. After her initial shock and pessimism at the child's birth, every positive achievement is likely to be given great emphasis, so that the standards she uses to evaluate intelligence are not necessarily those applied to normal children.

Above all, both Roskies (1972) and Voysey (1972a) have pointed out that mothers are likely to perceive intellectual ability and its expression in the type of school placement as constituting the children's major claim to normality. To question the child's intelligence may pose a major threat to the mother. Her emotional involvement in the question of where the child goes to school may be intense and, in the area of formal education, her tolerance for abnormality may, at least at this stage in the child's history, be limited.

*(ii) The doctor's perception of the main purpose of the meeting as being the systematic collection and rational evaluation of factual information about the child*

All too often the placement decision is not the end-product of a careful process of assessment in which medical officers, psychologists, teachers, social workers, administrators and above all the parents have made appropriate contributions, but of one short visit to the home by a medical officer or psychologist.

Such a person's time is limited; his main aim is to gather enough information to enable him to make an appropriate recommendation. This recommendation will, in many cases, amount to a final decision. Since he has become involved with handicapped children because they are *different* he is naturally likely to emphasise these differences, whereas the mother will tend to emphasise similarities with normal children. Having been trained to do so he will put greater reliance on test findings than on anecdotal evidence about the child's performance in 'everyday life', whereas the mother's orientation may be the reverse. In addition, as is true in the case of uncertain or unpleasant diagnoses, he may be reluctant to give parents information about the test findings. My own discussions with mothers suggest that in the great majority of cases professional—parent relationships as well as the parents' understanding of the child would be greatly improved if the professional explained more carefully to the mother the function of the test, and either at the time or in a follow-up session went over the findings and their implications with her. This is much more helpful to a mother than it is to be given vague and often misleading assurances about the child's potential.

*(iii) The mother's perception of education as providing a mode of compensation for the child*

It was mentioned earlier that mothers perceive education as providing one means by which a child can compensate for his disability. Here the extent of agreement with the doctor will depend on what type of school mothers see as offering the greater chances of compensation.

Once more, it is the association of the special schools with mental handicap that makes many parents unwilling to consider placement there. Thus the mother of a thalidomide girl in an industrial town states: 'A good education is important to her so that she can stand on her own feet. . . children who go to those schools are mentally backward . . . . I can't see how mixing with them would help her.' A farmworker and his wife with a spina bifida boy express the same viewpoint: 'We'd accept a special school if there weren't mentally handicapped children there. . . . I've got nothing against them — these things just happen . . . but we feel he needs really good education as he can't do manual work. We feel he wouldn't get this if he was with many other children of poorer ability.'

The following points made by Pringle and Fiddes (1970) about special school placement suggest that the mother's perception of the drawbacks of such placement may be realistic:

> Once in a special school there are a number of factors which are likely to depress still further the child's level of educational attainment: a shorter school day; fatigue due to lengthier journey to school; and probably most important of all there is also likely to be not only a lower standard of work (because there will be a high proportion of dull children) but probably also a lower level of expectation on the part of the teachers. For the majority of pupils this is entirely appropriate . . . but . . . the severely handicapped intelligent child may not always find himself sufficiently stimulated educationally.

*(iv) The doctor's perception of the alternatives available as regards school placement*

In his analysis of the sources of doctor—patient conflict Freidson (1971) draws attention to certain conflicts in perspective and interest that are 'built into the interaction and are likely to be present to some degree in every situation.' Doctors, for example, tend to handle cases conventionally while 'the patient wishes to be the exception to conventional rules'; and again the therapist (or doctor) tries to 'fit the single case into the convenience of organised practice while the patient struggles to gain a mode of management more specifically fitted to him as an individual'.

This conflict of perspectives can be seen when a doctor has to make recommendations about placement. He will be aware of the

Ministry of Education recommendation (Circular 276, 25 June 1954) that 'no handicapped child should be sent to a special school who can be satisfactorily educated in an ordinary school'. However, in the case of a 'marginal' child he is, understandably, more likely to 'handle the case conventionally' and to recommend placement in a special school than to attempt to make the sort of arrangements that might enable that child to attend an ordinary school. For most doctors the alternatives appear to be special school placement or placement in an ordinary class with no special help. Elsewhere a continuum of alternatives has been argued for (Anderson, 1973), including ordinary class placement with ancillary help, physical modifications to selected schools with the appointment of ancillary staff and the setting up of 'help clinics' or 'resource rooms', and a much greater extension of the special class system for disabled pupils.

This would of course demand much closer liaison between the doctors and the schools than has hitherto been the case, but it could mean a considerable reduction in the number of parents who felt that their children were simply being 'fitted into the convenience of organised practice.'

FACTORS AFFECTING BOTH STAGES OF THE INTERACTION

The mother brings two very important factors to the consultation about school placement, and they affect all aspects and stages of it. They are her perceptions and aspirations regarding the place of herself and her child, (i) in 'normal' society and (ii) in the community of the handicapped.

*(i) The mother's perception of the child's place in society*

For most parents of handicapped children the question of the child's place in society greatly influences the school placement decision. Most mothers hope that their children will function eventually as fully integrated members of the community: to some extent the mother's own social status is also involved, since, to the extent that mothers and children are viewed as a social unit, she may perceive the child's social failure as leading to a devaluation in her own status.

In Goffman's (1968) terms she carries a 'courtesy' stigma, that is a stigma attaching to a person simply through association with the stigmatised. At any consultation with a doctor, especially about school placement, the implications of the decision for social acceptance are therefore likely to be in the forefront of her mind.

'Society' is represented in a number of persons and a number of institutions: these will include the doctor who delivered the child, the family, neighbourhood friends, the hospital, the rehabilitation centre and the school. Roskies (1972) points out that 'society, in these various manifestations, plays a vital role in shaping the meaning and course of events', but that what usually happens is that 'the needs of the mother, child, and society, rather than working in harmony become embroiled in a complex conflict of interests'. When a child who is different from the normal is born, the *meaning* of this difference has to be supplied by society, 'which, validly or invalidly, considers physical abnormality as a form of social deviance and which, as a consequence, has no defined place in the existing social structure for these children. . . . We need to recognize the fact that the problem of the handicapped child is caused as much by society as by his own deficiency or his mother's reaction to it, and the solution must include all three parties.'

There is no doubt that most mothers (and, in theory, most professionals) perceive ordinary school placement as likely to facilitate society's acceptance of the child or, at worst, the child's ability to cope with society's ambivalence. Some mothers in my own study emphasised the former: one stated, 'It's terribly important for her to mix with ordinary children and to be at school where all the local people know her. They treat her just like anyone else.' Other mothers stressed the child's need to adapt to society: 'The younger they live with normal people, the quicker they'll adapt. They're always going to get comments, and the younger they accept it the better.'

In her communications with a doctor a mother may frequently try to enlist him as an ally to help her to handle social conflict. However, the vast majority of doctors are oriented to patients and illness, and have neither the training nor the inclination to take on this role. Moreover, lack of sociological and psychiatric training means that they are unlikely to have much theoretical knowledge of interpersonal relationships.

*(ii) The mother's perception of her own and her child's relationship with other handicapped people*

In a study of mothers of mentally retarded children Birenbaum (1970) points out that 'friendships with others who are stigmatized do not support a normal-appearing . . . life' and that in general mothers participated in the organised world of mental retardation only when they could see this to be of some specific use to the child.

In my own study considerable variation was found in the extent to which mothers of physically handicapped children wished to identify themselves and their children with other parents and children in a similar situation. There can be no doubt that they tended to be extremely anxious to avoid identification of their children with the mentally retarded. In Roskies's words, 'any suggestion which links the two is threatening, as it represents a denial of the child's major claim to normality'. Thus many mothers were opposed to special school placement because they believed that there were 'mentally handicapped', 'retarded' or 'backward' children in the schools for the physically handicapped (which is of course to some extent true). One mother felt that 'everyone would be looking at her [child] and saying "she's a bit simple", when they saw the special buses'. Others thought that the child's self-image would be affected, for example that the child would 'get an inferiority complex' or 'be more self-conscious' or that such placement would 'plant in his mind that he's different'.

Mothers whose children have minimal handicaps naturally have high expectations that the child will 'pass' in the normal community. They are likely to be especially anxious to avoid identification with the handicapped community, and even a slight setback, such as a doctor's casual reference to the possibility of special schooling, may have serious connotations and may give rise to misperceptions. One mother whose child had a very minor post-thalidomide deformity (affecting only two fingers) reported that shortly before the child started school she took her to see the registrar, who 'had a file of papers for the handicapped school in front of him'. According to the mother, 'I refused to let her go, and that was the end of it.'

Where the handicap is an 'invisible' one such as incontinence, there is often the same hope that the child will 'pass' in the normal community. A mother whose child had internal congenital deformities with resultant incontinence stated, 'I was distressed [when a special school was suggested]. . . . You see the special transport coming with mongols and all. He's forward in his mind. I could imagine him sitting there thinking "there's something wrong with them, there must be something wrong with me." After all, they're kids with funny faces and irons.'

IMPROVING MOTHER—DOCTOR INTERACTIONS

Various factors have been considered that might have an adverse effect upon mother—doctor interactions when a decision has to be made about the school placement of a handicapped child. Some conflict between mothers and doctors may be inevitable.

However the situation could be improved and Figure 2 suggests how this might be done. The figure incorporates three important new features. Firstly, both mother and doctor (or other professional, such as an educational psychologist) are represented as bringing various needs and expectancies to their first interaction, these being the factors discussed in the preceding sections. An awareness of the strength of these factors could often lead to better mother—doctor interactions; to achieve this, improved training of professionals in the management of chronic handicap is needed.

A second way in which this diagram differs from the earlier one is that at least two (rather than one) mother—doctor meetings are proposed, the aim of the first being the proposal of a *possible* solution requiring further exploration rather than a final decision. This would have the great advantage of giving both parties, particularly the parents, time to think over the information gained from the first meeting and to discuss the proposed placement. Knowledge that no final decisions would be taken during this first interaction should make the situation less stressful for the mother, and thus facilitate both stages A (relationship formation) and B (the giving and receiving of information).

The third important feature now incorporated is the school which has been suggested. Arrangements could be made for the mother and the doctor (or other professional) to visit the school separately to discuss the placement proposal first with the head and then, if the head is willing to consider the placement, with the person likely to be

*Figure 2*    *The mother—doctor interaction — revised version*

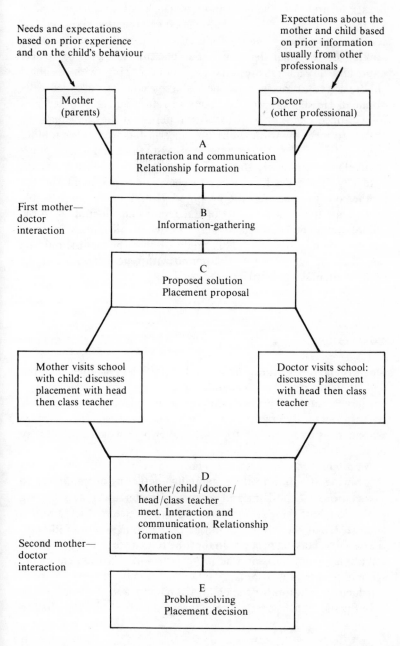

the child's class teacher. It is also important that the child should see the school and meet the head and class teacher. It may be preferable for the mother to see the head alone first and then to make a second visit with the child. The doctor's visit to the school *prior* to the making of the final decision about placement is also extremely important. Teachers are anxious about coping with disabled children, yet at present teacher—doctor contacts are generally minimal. Heads, too, are less likely to refuse outright to accept a handicapped child, at least for a trial period, if they have had the chance to meet the professional(s) concerned as well as the mother and child beforehand, and have been assured of ongoing support particularly in the early stages of placement.

Ideally, if the head and class teacher on the one hand and the mother on the other felt the proposed placement was in principle acceptable, the separate visits of the doctor and the mother to the school would be followed by stage D, where all parties met and decided about placement. This might be that the child should be placed in the school for a trial period with regular reviews of the appropriateness of the placement.

CONCLUSION

Doctors and other professionals working with handicapped children and their parents are generally highly motivated and deeply concerned about the welfare of their clients. Despite this, parent—doctor interactions are frequently unsatisfactory. School placement is by no means the only matter over which conflict may arise.

An attempt has been made to clarify some of the reasons for this by drawing attention to the potentially conflicting perceptions and expectations of mothers and doctors. Greater awareness among professionals of these factors could help to reduce conflict, and it is suggested that the school should be brought much more fully into the decision-making process. In the long run, more time spent on the initial placement decision and more systematic involvement of the schools (especially ordinary schools) should provide a more satisfactory solution for the child, the parents and the teachers.

In the past it has generally been the handicapped who have had to adapt to society. There are many signs, expressed for example in a growing militancy among the disabled themselves, that in future society will be expected to be more accommodating and also that the consumer or the consumer's parents will have a stronger voice in deciding what form special services should take. It is within this context that these comments and suggestions concerning mother—doctor interactions are offered.

# 4 Professional Autonomy and Client Exclusion: a Study in ENT Clinics

## by Michael Bloor

### INTRODUCTION

Freidson has pointed to functional autonomy — independence from lay evaluation and control — as an identifying characteristic of professional work: functional autonomy is 'the test of professional status' (Freidson, 1971, p. 84). Thus, Freidson designates functional autonomy as a *structural* property of a particular class of occupations. However, his analysis also implies that functional autonomy may be generated in the process of professional—client interaction. The location of functional autonomy in the process of interaction is perhaps most clearly evident in Freidson's discussion of Evans-Pritchard's description of witch-doctoring among the Azande (Freidson, 1971, pp. 6—11). This chapter is concerned with functional autonomy as an aspect of *process*. Using data on the interaction between ENT (ear, nose and throat) specialists and parents of children referred for assessment for possible adeno-tonsillectomy ('Ts and As') I shall try to show how certain routine assessment practices employed by specialists in ENT clinics may affect parents' ability to influence the outcome of consultations; functional autonomy can be both embodied in and facilitated by specialists' routine work practices. I shall argue that doctors' autonomy may not be a universal feature of medical encounters, and that an important determinant of the degree of autonomy that a particular doctor may possess in a certain setting may be the character of the work practices he routinely adopts to manage everyday medical tasks.

## THE DATA[1]

Following a period of preliminary study and discussion with the specialists involved, systematic observations were carried out in the course of nearly five hundred consultations at the outpatient clinics of eleven ENT specialists. The patients were all children under fifteen, newly referred to the clinic for assessment for possible adeno-tonsillectomy. In all cases, at least one responsible adult (usually the mother) was present during the consultation. The parent—doctor exchanges reported here were recorded manually without the assistance of a tape recorder, and I am confident that they are substantially accurate reconstructions of the exchanges.[2] Some additional material was collected in the course of tape recorded semi-structured interviews with the same specialists.

## ON SPECIALISTS' ROUTINES

Assessment of children for possible adeno-tonsillectomy is a routine event for ENT specialists. The constantly recurring need to assess such children day in day out, year in year out ensures that the specialist's clinic world approximates to that described by Schutz as 'a world of routine activities' (Schutz, 1970, pp. 138—41), a world populated by familiar complaints to which familiar investigatory procedures can be applied to yield up familiar findings which imply familiar forms of therapeutic intervention.[3] This familiarity may occasionally be disrupted by the intrusion of the unexpected, but over time many disruptions will themselves become familiar and will be handled in a familiar way, so that novel situations, where the specialists feels his responses to be problematic, will become rarer and rarer occurrences. The routine nature of much clinic work is not solely an observer's construct, it is an interpretation shared by the specialists themselves; as one of them wryly put it, 'I ought to make a record.'

I shall designate the familiar tried and tested recipes employed by specialists in processing children through their clinics by the generic term 'routines', following Fletcher's observational work on doctor—patient interaction (Fletcher, 1974). These various routines are not only a mechanism whereby a high degree of consistency in each specialist's practice obtains over a large number of encounters;

they also serve to render specialists' disposal decisions unproblematic: by following his familiar routines the specialist sets in train a course of events through which he may unproblematically give assent to one of his stock of familiar forms of therapeutic intervention.

Decision rules and search procedures and specialists' modes of clinic organisation are examples of kinds of routines studied here. By a specialist's decision rules I mean those informal, pragmatic rules-of-thumb concerning which symptoms and signs the specialist feels to be typically minimally acceptable for allocating children to the various alternative forms of therapeutic intervention at his disposal (the term 'decision rule' is taken from Scheff, 1963). By a specialist's search procedures I mean those standard investigatory routines the specialist needs to operationalise his various decision rules (the term 'search procedure' is taken from Douglas, 1967). By a specialist's mode of clinic organisation I mean such clinic features as the seating arrangements in the consultation room, and the availability of access to certain investigatory procedures such as audiometric assessment and X-ray. Certain of the routines followed by specialists will not have been adopted free of external constraints; some aspects of specialists' modes of clinic organisation form examples of such routines.

A specialist's routines may be related to his autonomy of function in two analytically distinct ways. In the first place, there is a sense in which their sum is the *embodiment* of his functional autonomy. They serve to orchestrate consultations according to specialists', not parents', purposes.[4] They may have the effect of excluding the parent from effective participation in the disposal decision simply through their structuring of the consultation without regard for the parent's purposes. Thus, while the doctor may have a diffuse, culturally approved 'right' to legislate by fiat in health and illness, the totality of his routines are the practical embodiment of his dominance in the medical encounter.

Yet in addition to the above general sense in which routines embody specialists' functional autonomy they also, in a more particular sense, *facilitate* specialists' autonomy. Routines can be seen not as just simply excluding parents by structuring consultations according to specialists' purposes, but as actively denying parents any potential influence. This process of active denial has been characterised by Lemert (1968) as 'the dynamics of exclusion'. Lemert depicted a number of interactional routines by which ego may exclude alter from exercising influence, viz. patronising, evasion, 'humouring', guiding conversation on to selected topics, under-reaction and silence. In the ENT clinic a number of different routines were employed by different specialists which would have the effect of contributing to specialists' autonomy.[5] The nature of the routines employed affects how far the parent is excluded from possible participation in the disposal decision, and the autonomy of a particular specialist's decisions. Some routines will have the effect, other things being equal, of excluding parents more fully than others, and others may serve to enlarge the scope for parental participation. Since specialists' routines differed markedly (though a number of routines were common to more than one specialist), it is not surprising that inter-specialist differences were observed in the degree of exclusion of parents from possible participation in the disposal decision. In what follows various specialists' routines are compared to show their differential contribution to specialists' functional autonomy. For descriptive purposes the routines are divided into three categories. First, there are inhibitory routines which may have the effect of denying parents recourse to actions that might influence case disposal, or that of deterring parents from such activities. Second, there are reactive routines which may nullify parental actions that might otherwise influence the specialist in favour of a surgical disposal. Finally, there are reconciliatory routines which may reconcile reluctant parents to a surgical disposal.

Before beginning this comparative description it is appropriate to consider the various channels of potential parent influence over case disposal.

CHANNELS OF PARENTAL INFLUENCE

Two channels of potential parent influence over case disposal can be isolated. One is the indirect influence that may occur through the parental history. The specialist's disposal decision concerning a particular child may vary with the nature of the parent's account of the biophysical events in the child's illness career. However, the potential for such indirect influence will vary between specialists, and is a function of their routines. Obviously the potential for such influence on the disposal decision is greater where the specialist's decision rules emphasise the importance of the parent history relative to the examination, or indeed relative to the GP's history. A second factor regulating the potential for influence is the specific form of the search procedures used in the history-taking. The search procedures of Dr A can serve as an illustration.

Dr A wanted to establish how extensively a child had been troubled before deciding whether or not to list him for Ts and As. On different occasions he asked either how long attacks had been suffered, or he tried to ascertain the frequency of attacks, or he tried to ascertain both, or simply asked if the child had suffered 'a lot' of trouble.

| | |
|---|---|
| *Dr A:* | A lot of sore throats? |
| *Mother:* | Yes. |
| *Dr A:* | [examining the child] When was the last time? |
| *Mother:* | About three weeks ago. |
| *Dr A:* | He's got glands there. Do they come up with these attacks? |
| *Mother:* | Yes. |
| *Dr A:* | Congested-looking tonsils. |
| *Mother:* | He's got an awful runny nose at the moment. |
| *Dr A:* | Mouth open pretty well all the time is it? |
| *Mother:* | Yes. |
| *Dr A:* | Noisy sleeper? |
| *Mother:* | Yes. |
| *Dr A:* | Appetite? |
| *Mother:* | It's better now than it used to be. It used to be poor. |

The examination revealed large, congested tonsils, large glands and discharge from the nose. The child was listed for Ts and As.

It would seem that merely to ask whether the child has suffered 'a lot' of trouble may allow the parent greater potential influence over disposal, than would collecting information about the length and frequency of attacks. In the former case the specialist must rely on the parent's assessment of the troublesomeness of symptoms, while in the latter, though dependent on the parent's account of the symptomatology, he may draw his own conclusions on their relative troublesomeness. This distinction is important because at least some specialists view a certain amount of tonsillar infection as 'normal'.

The following exchange illustrates this divergence between expert and lay assessments of troublesomeness:

*Dr F:*   What's the trouble?
*Mother:*   He's bothered by tonsillitis a lot.
*Dr F:*   Doctor [the GP] says he isn't. Which is the truth?
*Mother:*   Well he had a bad attack and then it seemed to keep coming back.
*Dr F:*   Yes but that would be just one attack really. Has he had any trouble with the ears?

In addition to the potential for indirect influence afforded by specialist routines that emphasise the importance of the history supplied by the parent, a second, and more direct, channel of potential parent influence lies in opening up what might be termed the 'hidden agenda' of clinic consultations.

Specialists did not explicitly recognise that the rationale for many consultations was to assess whether or not Ts and As was indicated: they focused consultations on patients' symptoms and signs rather than on a discussion of possible disposals. Thus one channel of potential parent influence lies in making the hidden agenda explicit, in engaging in activities that will inaugurate a discussion of the appropriate form of therapeutic intervention for their child. As Scheff puts it, 'the more explicit the agenda of the transaction, the more control the client gets over the resulting definition of the situation', or outcome (Scheff, 1968, p. 16).

Once again, though, the potential for influence through opening up the hidden agenda is a function of the particular specialist routines employed. Thus, a number of specialists began their consultations with an invitation to the parent to describe their child's problem; e.g., 'What's the trouble, mum?' Such routines provide parents with a conversational opportunity right at the outset of the consultation to open up the agenda. Likewise, those specialists whose decision rules emphasised the importance of the parent's history also tended to provide more conversational opportunities for opening up the agenda than those whose decision rules emphasised the examination findings, and whose history-taking was correspondingly briefer.

These descriptions of specialists' routines can of course be seen as evidence *against* the argument that routines serve to maintain specialists' functional autonomy. However, each of the routines described that permit parental influences of a direct or indirect nature are countervailed by other routines employed by the same specialist on the same cases. Although each of the routines described would tend, by itself, to reduce the specialist's autonomy of function by permitting parents to influence the disposal decision, their effect is nullified by other routines. Thus, Dr A was described as employing a search procedure (in seeking to establish how extensively a child had been troubled) such that the specialist would take over the parent's assessment of troublesomeness for his own. However, this is offset by the relatively large part the examination findings play in his disposal decision. The patient in this consultation had, on examination, evidence of tonsillar infection. Where the parental history of sore throats was not corroborated by examination, Dr A's questioning concerning the troublesomeness of the symptoms was both more extensive and more concerned with quantitative information in the history. What Garfinkel (1967) calls the degree of 'tolerable error' in the history-taking was reduced. This is illustrated by the following excerpt from a case where the examination findings were innocuous.

| | |
|---|---|
| *Dr A:* | What age are you? |
| *Child:* | Eleven. |
| *Dr. A:* | How long has he been having these sore throats? |
| *Mother:* | It's been off and on for quite some time. |
| *Dr A:* | Yes, but how long? |
| *Mother:* | Four or five years. |
| *Dr A:* | Two or three times a year? |
| *Mother:* | Yes. |

Likewise, routines that encouraged parental behaviour which might open up the agenda were also nullified by other routines. Specialists employed reactive routines in response to such parental behaviour, and this had the effect of maintaining their autonomy unimpaired.

A detailed description of those routines that served to maintain specialists' autonomy is provided below, but first it is necessary that one routine (employed only by Dr B) be detailed since this constitutes an exception, in so far as it granted a substantial measure of control over disposal to parents under certain circumstances.

Once Dr B had established to his satisfaction the symptoms of the children he saw, then, if he recognised that some form of active intervention was necessary but surgery was not an immediate ethical necessity, he would offer the parents a choice. He would agree either to put the child on the waiting list for surgery or to deal with the child conservatively by recommending long-term chemotherapy and reviewing the case.

*Dr B:*     Does he get lots of sore throats?
*Mother:*   Yes, and colds and a runny nose.
*Dr B:*     But he gets sore throats?
*Mother:*   Yes, he's had tonsillitis a few times.
*Dr B:*     Are they getting any better?
*Mother:*   Oh, no!
*Dr B:*     How long has he been getting sore throats?
*Mother:*   Since he was about six months.
*Dr B:*     And he's 4 now?
*Mother:*   Yes.
*Dr B:*     So that's 3½ years he's had them?
*Mother:*   Yes.
*Dr B:*     Does he snore at all?
*Mother:*   Yes.
*Dr B:*     Have his ears ever burst or discharged?
*Mother:*   No.
            [Dr B examines the child.]
*Dr B:*     If we take his tonsils out that should put an end to his sore throats. How do you feel about that? If we do nothing he'll probably grow out of it but I don't know when. How do you feel about it?
*Mother:*   Well I'd prefer it if you did take them out because it helped my other boy.
            [Dr B lists the child for Ts and As]

Dr B was the only specialist in the sample explicitly prepared to surrender his functional autonomy to parents who favoured a surgical disposal in certain circumstances. This was both intentional (in the sense that Dr B felt it was proper to take parents' wishes into account in such cases) and the consequence of particular routines, rather than being unintended and the consequence of parental activities that may have been designed to influence the disposal decision. Of course, not all parents were prepared to be placed in this position of being arbiter of their child's disposal: a few returned the ball to the specialist's court; one told him, 'You're the doctor'.

## INHIBITORY ROUTINES

Inhibitory routines are those modes of clinic organisation, decision rules and search procedures that may deter parents from opening up the agenda and deny them the opportunity of a large measure of indirect influence through the history. Consider first the following three routines of Dr C as examples of ways in which the mode of clinic organisation can be seen as a species of inhibitory routine.

In the consultation room Dr C sat directly opposite the child and took the history during his examination, with the parent seated to one side. The lack of face-to-face contact with the specialist and the air the specialist may give of being absorbed in his examination may make parents reluctant to intrude with unsolicited remarks. In addition, Dr C's opening remarks were addressed to the child: 'Hello. Have a sit beside me' (pointing to the chair in front of him). He ignored the mother who was directed to a chair by a nurse. Thus, the usual parent—child status hierarchy was reversed, and the mother was treated as an appendage of the child. Finally, in many cases Dr C's disposal decision was not taken at the time of the consultation but only after he had received the results of certain investigations (e.g. X-rays, audiograms, etc.) and the parent was informed of the eventual decision by the GP. This distance between the disposal decision and the consultation both reduces the possibility of a parent-initiated discussion of disposal, and may also emphasise to the parent the specialist's functional autonomy.[6]

Not only clinic organisation but also decision rules adopted by specialists may militate against parents' introducing the topic of disposals and may restrict the opportunities for indirect influence through the history. Thus Dr D, for certain categories of cases, assumed that the arrival of a child at his clinic, the fact of referral of itself, indicated the likelihood of a history requiring listing for Ts and As (as he put it, 'if a child's been sent up, there must be some history'). If this assumption was confirmed, as it nearly always was, by the examination findings, then the outcome was decided regardless of the history given by the parents. As a consequence the parental contribution to many consultations, and hence the potential for influence, was minimal. For example, a GP's letter described a 'long history of recurring nasal, ear and URTI' (upper respiratory tract infection) and a 'tendency to bronchospasm'. The GP wondered if tonsillectomy was indicated. The total history was as follows:

| | |
|---|---|
| *Dr D:* | She gets colds and sore throats and things does she? |
| *Mother:* | She's never complained of a sore throat. She's just very thick with it. |
| | [On examination Dr D found 'enormous congested tonsils', 'very big' glands, and a 'thick discharge' from the nose, and the child was listed for Ts and As.] |

Likewise, the nature of the search procedures may serve to inhibit parents from raising the topic of disposals. If the GP letter gave Dr D what he regarded as an adequate case for tonsillectomy, he confined history-taking to cross-checking the GP's report with the parent and to checking for additional symptoms of adenoid enlargement. This procedure allows specialists to frame their questions to parents in forms that demand specific rather than elaborated replies, and so provide little in the way of a conversational opening for parents to raise the topic of disposal. Specialists may also frame their questions in a similar manner without the benefit of information from the GP (i.e., they may make statements about the child's symptomatology and invite parents to confirm or deny them), with the same inhibitory effect on parents. The following consultation conducted by Dr H contains examples of both types of question.

The GP's letter referred to '. . . a number of episodes of upper respiratory infection in the past' and to the fact that during his penultimate attack the child required admission to hospital. The child's enlarged tonsils were also mentioned. The GP felt that the child would benefit from Ts and As.

| | |
|---|---|
| *Dr H:* | How old is he? |
| *Mother:* | 19 months. |
| *Dr H:* | He's had two bad attacks? |
| *Mother:* | Yes. |
| *Dr H:* | He's fevered? |
| *Mother:* | Yes. |
| *Dr H:* | And he came into hospital with one of them? |
| *Mother:* | Yes. |
| *Dr H:* | In between times he's all right? |
| *Mother:* | Yes. |
| *Dr H:* | He eats his food? |
| *Mother:* | Yes, fine. |

*Dr H:*     He hasn't had ear trouble?
*Mother:*   No.

Search procedures adopted by specialists may also severely limit the potential for indirect parental influence through the parental history. Thus, Dr E employed search procedures that elicited quantitative data on the extent and severity of a child's symptoms, and so allowed him to draw his own conclusions about their extensiveness and severity. Dr E also often cross-checked parental accounts and 'normalised' children's symptoms (i.e. reinterpreting symptoms to parents as manifesting 'normal' child behaviour, or a 'normal' degree of morbidity), and thus discouraged what he regarded as exaggerated parental assessments of a child's symptoms. He emphasised his right to a monopoly on the interpretation of symptoms. For example:

*Mother:*   She breathes through her mouth, it's [the nose] always blocked.
*Dr E:*     All the time? I just ask because she hasn't been breathing through her mouth since she came into the room.
*Mother:*   It's odd times, mostly at night.
*Dr E:*     Well, I wouldn't worry too much about that. Half the adult population breathe through their mouths when they sleep and we don't suggest surgical remedies for them. I think children should have the same rights.

⋮

*Dr E:*     What's the trouble?
*Mother:*   He gets sore throats and sometimes he gets sore ears too. It's every month he has a sore throat.
*Dr E:*     How long has this been going on for?
*Mother:*   Since he started school in September.
*Dr E:*     Is he in bed when he's off school?
*Mother:*   Yes.
*Dr E:*     How long is he in bed for?
*Mother:*   Just a couple of days.
*Dr E:*     How many attacks has he had in all?
*Mother:*   Six.
*Dr E:*     Just a minute. Six months since September, one a month. That's right. This earache, is it just with the sore throats?

*Mother:*   Yes.

*Dr E:*   [to author]: It's probably just reactive [examining the child]. One tiny gland on each side. Tonsils large but quite clean. Nose is all right. Timpanic membranes all right — it's probably just reactive as I thought,
[to mother] He's not getting really bad sore throats and an awful lot of kids get this when they start school. . . .

Finally, one inhibitory routine employed by a number of specialists was the production of a short 'account' (cf. Scott and Lyman, 1968) for their disposal decisions. Such accounts were more likely to be used when specialists had decided against an immediate surgical disposal. Parents who might wish to query the disposal decision must then directly challenge the socially legitimated expertise of the specialist.

One of the specialists who habitually provided accounts for his conservative disposals would explain his decision to parents in terms of the examination findings, although it was normally the child's history that was the most influential factor in his disposal decision. In one case he wrote to the GP saying, '. . . I feel his troubles are really not very frequent or severe and one should treat him conservatively for the time being', while he told the parents: 'The tonsils are not that bad, I think we could afford to wait a little while and see how he gets along.' Conceivably, parents would feel less able to query the implications of examination findings than the specialist's assessment of the history.

REACTIVE ROUTINES

Some specialists' routines allowed parents relatively more scope for activities that might open up the hidden agenda. However, specialists whose routines did allow parents to raise the topic of disposals also employed reactive routines which served to nullify such potential parental influence.

The lack of impact on disposals of parents' opening up the agenda may be partially attributable to the manner in which parents raised the topic of disposals. I observed no instance of parents baldly stating their opinion that the tonsils should be removed;[7] rather, parents would raise the topic in a way that avoided a direct challenge, and would maintain deference to the specialist's socially legitimated expertise.[8] Thus, the most common form of topic-raising was the simple inquiry as to whether the specialist thought tonsillectomy was required, and another common form was to mention the GP's diagnosis or his feeling that tonsillectomy might be necessary.

In these cases specialists' reactive routines were able to enforce speedy closure. Where the GP was invoked, specialists would return the encounter to a discussion of symptoms: 'Well let me put it this way — why did you take him to the doctor in the first place?' Where parents inquired about disposal, specialists would either ignore the parental invitation to discuss disposals or they would provide a short account; e.g.:

| | |
|---|---|
| *Dr F:* | No ear trouble, no tonsils trouble [contradicting an earlier parental diagnosis]. All right! |
| *Mother:* | She doesn't need her tonsils out? |
| *Dr F:* | Not at present, no. [To child] Bye-bye. |

| | |
|---|---|
| *Mother:* | And the tonsils are all right as well? |
| *Dr G:* | They're quite big . . . |
| *Mother:* | Yes, they're awfully big. |
| *Dr G:* | . . . but if they're not causing any trouble it would be better to leave them in. They'll go down as she gets older. |
| *Mother:* | Oh, they will? |
| *Dr G:* | Yes. |
| *Mother:* | Oh, that's all right then. |

RECONCILIATORY ROUTINES

So far I have described those specialist routines that ensured that parents were unable to influence specialists in favour of a surgical disposal. The position is somewhat different where parents may be reluctant for their children to undergo surgery. Various routines may either facilitate or inhibit the expression of parental reluctance to sanction surgery, like those that affected the possibility of parents opening up the agenda, but when parental doubts *are* expressed, routine responses of specialists take on a rather different character from the reactive routines described above.

A detailed analysis of why specialists' routines should differ where parents expressed doubts about sanctioning surgery is not attempted here, but the following can be said about the various 'problem relevances' (Emerson, 1969, pp. 83—4), which specialists may see as present in such situations. Briefly, the 'problem relevances', not all of them articulated by all specialists, are these.

Failure to operate where indicated may condemn a child to unnecessary subsequent morbidity, while on the other hand postponement of a final decision on whether or not to operate is unlikely to have a permanently deleterious effect on the child.[9] Also, continuance of recurrent morbidity may make the parents more favourably disposed to surgery at some future date; in the event of serious post-operative complications or death a parent who has only reluctantly agreed to the operation is more likely to have recourse to the complaints procedure than other parents, and a parent can block a surgical disposal by refusing to sign the operation consent form.

There is a wide variation between specialists in the use of routines that may facilitate or inhibit the expression of parental reluctance to sanction surgery. At one extreme Dr B explicitly places the disposal decision in the hands of the parents in certain cases, and Dr G, when faced with a patient whom he feels requires surgery, routinely explains that surgery would be justified and asks 'are you willing?' At the other extreme Dr C sometimes fails to communicate any disposal decision to the parent, and Dr A often only communicates in an oblique way his decision to operate. Dr A's lack of explicitness in communicating a surgical disposal is related to a wish not to alarm the child.

Further considerable inter-specialist differences occur in routine responses to parents' *expressed* reluctance.[10] When Dr G obtained what he took to be a negative response to his question 'are you willing', he immediately discharged the child. Dr E, in contrast, contested the decision with parents, and drew attention to his own expertise and authority, so that those who wished to avoid surgery for their child had to reject that expertise and authority.

*Dr E:*  We'll have to get this wax removed — that's one thing. She may have catarrh behind it. I don't know. Also she's got an awful lot of glands down there [points to child's neck] and I think she should have her tonsils out.

| | |
|---|---|
| *Mother:* | Well, do you really think . . . ? I don't want her to unless . . . ? |
| *Dr E:* | OK it's up to you [not said dismissively]. |
| | There are two different problems here. She's got this deafness and she's also got these swollen glands. |
| *Mother:* | What will it entail, these glands? |
| *Dr E:* | It's a sign she's going to have trouble with her tonsils. My experience over many years is that she's going to have trouble. Now, she's got to come into hospital with the ears. Why not have them both done at the same time? It's quite possible that she has abscesses in these glands and she'll have to have them opened. It's your decision, but I would strongly advise it. |
| *Mother:* | You would. |
| *Dr E:* | Yes. Of course I wouldn't say she should have them out unless I strongly advise it. |
| *Mother:* | Very well then. |

A number of specialists took an intermediate position and elected to review in the belief that parents would eventually overcome their doubts. One told parents to discuss the matter with their GP, and wrote to the GP explaining his belief that surgery was indicated.

No specialist routines were proof against the eventualities of parents getting in touch with the hospital authorities and saying that they'd decided against surgery (I recorded two such instances), or of parents simply failing to deliver up their children on the prescribed admission date.

CONCLUSION

Clinic consultations are structured by sets of specialist routines, some routines being employed by more than one specialist. Specialists' routines may either allow considerable scope for parental participation in disposal decisions, or effectively exclude parents from such participation. The former were normally employed by specialists in conjunction with other routines which nullified any potential parental influence on disposals. Thus, specialists' routines may be said to *produce* specialists' functional autonomy in everyday clinic encounters.

However, specialist autonomy was not a universal feature of all the clinic encounters studied. Exceptions occurred when some specialists were confronted with parents who were reluctant to sanction surgery, and one specialist (Dr B) who in certain cases would routinely leave the final decision to the child's parents.

It would therefore appear that, while functional autonomy may receive general social endorsement as a characteristic of professional work, the extent to which it is manifest in everyday professional activities varies, and is dependent on a number of forces which may favour or militate against the processual production of professional dominance. Undoubtedly, one such set of forces concerns the clinical and organisational setting for the medical encounter, and the various resources and constraints that clients and professionals may feel this setting affords them or imposes on them. But whether or not functional autonomy is processually generated in an encounter may also depend on the various routine practices employed by the professional in the accomplishment of everyday tasks.

NOTES

1   The data on which this chapter is based were collected in the course of a study of ENT practice financed by the Medical Research Council.

2   The manual recording of conversations clearly involves the recorder in the unthinking translation of utterances from a spoken sense to a written sense. For example, false starts, hesitations while the speaker gropes for a word and so on tend to be excluded, and grammatical sense is unthinkingly imposed. Thus, manually recorded transcripts can never reproduce conversations with the same accuracy as verbatim transcripts taken from tape recordings.

3   It is not being suggested here that the specialist's knowledge is of an identical character to that habitual or routinised knowledge ideal — typically depicted by Schutz and Luckmann and sub-divided by them into 'skills', 'useful knowledge' and 'knowledge of recipes' (Schutz and Luckmann, 1974, pp. 105—11). By describing the specialist's clinic world as 'a world of routine activities', I am not postulating an exact correspondence between specialist's knowledge and any one of these pure types described by Schutz and Luckmann, but that the specialist's knowledge contains important elements of habitual knowledge. As Schutz and Luckmann put it, 'Routinisation can . . . enter into other provinces of finite meaning-structure. . . . There is habitual knowledge in scientific thinking, even if this cannot be legitimated in terms of scientific theory' (pp. 110—111).

4   Of course, parents' purposes need not necessarily conflict with those of the specialists. For example, some parents may simply wish to facilitate the specialists' task in reaching whatever decision on disposal he deems advisable. Likewise, parents' purposes may be subject to modification as the encounter proceeds and eventually come to harmonise with the specialist's purposes. This process of modification of parents' purposes may be influenced by the particular routines adopted by the specialist, so that a coalescence of client and professional purposes may emerge. Scheff (1968) has called this a 'negotiation process', though it may occur without

either party viewing the situation as one of negotiation and without parental purposes being necessarily well defined at the outset. Indeed, the 'change' in parental purposes may simply be a change in the clarity of definition of those purposes in the course of the consultation: specialists' routines may, in some instances, instil in parents the purpose of aiding the specialist in reaching whatever disposal decision he deems necessary where no clear parental purpose existed before.

5    It should not be assumed that all the specialists in the sample always employed the depicted routines with the intention of facilitating their dominance of encounters; this assumption would not be justified from the data. Rather the point being made here is that the depicted routines may have *the effect* of maintaining specialists' autonomy, regardless of specialists' particular purposes at hand. It is my intention simply to describe specialists' routines and their relation to the production of functional autonomy. Clearly it is not possible to do this without some reference to the motives of the specialists and the imputations specialists make of the motives of the parents. However, I wish merely to refer to specialists' motives and imputations *en passant*, since motivation in the encounters appears (as one would expect in situations where the actor is not normally required to account for his behaviour) so complex as to require a paper to itself.

6    It is not the case that this distancing of the disposal decision from the consultation is an inevitable consequence of the specialist commissioning these investigative procedures: at other clinics I observed, arrangements existed which resulted in specialists assessing the results of their commissioned investigations and deciding on a disposal in the presence of parents.

7    Perhaps the closest any parent came to such a bald statement of belief occurred in the following exchange:

*Dr F:*    Now, what's the trouble?
*Mother:*    He seems to have permanently enlarged tonsils, his speech is adenoidal, he pokes at his food. His sister had the same trouble until the tonsils were removed.

8    A parallel can be drawn here with the 'hinting' techniques Edgerton (1965) describes as characterising native behaviour when seeking access to resources held by whites.

9    Specialists reported that they would be more likely to pursue the matter of a surgical disposal and would pursue it with more force if faced with parental reluctance to sanction surgery where the child in question was suffering from otitis media, a disorder that can — if untreated — result in permanent hearing loss.

10    The relatively small number of cases I observed where parents expressed doubts about a surgical disposal necessarily means that my description of specialists' routine responses is drawn in part from interviews with specialists as well as from observation.

# 5  A Linguistic Description of Doctor–Patient Interviews

## by Malcolm Coulthard and Margaret Ashby

### INTRODUCTION

In 1935 J. R. Firth wrote that in 'the study of conversation . . . we shall find the key to a better understanding of what language really is and how it works' (Firth, 1957), but serious work on how language is organised into meaningful patterns above the sentence has only just begun. The research[1] described here is part of an ongoing attempt to develop a linguistic theory and description of verbal interaction through a study of the language used in a number of socially defined situations: classrooms, doctor—patient interviews, committee meetings and television discussion programmes.

Verbal interaction can be approached from a number of different disciplines: the social scientist may be interested in how it displays social processes and social structure; the grammarian in the stylistic, dialectal or idiolectal features. For us the interesting aspect of verbal interaction is the socio-linguistic organisation, the way in which grammatical units such as sentences and clauses are used functionally by speakers to achieve social ends.

We are interested in the structure of all forms of spoken discourse ranging from desultory conversation between two people of equal status to highly formal situations such as debates and trial by jury. We are interested in how turns to speak are distributed or negotiated, how topics are introduced and closed, what verbal strategies participants use to achieve their ends, how successive utterances are related and how individual utterances are interpreted as having a given meaning in a given context.

Our early attempts to analyse casual conversation were not particularly successful. Equal participants negotiate in subtle and complex ways for the right to speak and the right to control the direction of the discourse or introduce new topics. Conversation is a joint production, and while one speaker may indicate to the others the way in which he wants the discourse to go, if the others do not accept his lead there is not a lot he can do about it — speakers talk about what interests them and when something ceases or fails to interest them they change the topic. In order to reduce some of the variation and complexity we decided to choose situations in which institutional definitions constrain the purposes and goals of the interaction and the roles of the participants. In such studies the discourse structure is more obvious and repetitive.

Our focus on discourse in specific situations is thus an heuristic one. The doctor—patient interview was selected partly in order to contrast with the three other situations on such dimensions as number of participants, presence or absence of an audience, equality of status of participants, and partly because it was fairly easy to collect the data. Our categorisation of the interview as a situation type was again heuristic and based on lay definitions of 'different' situations. We are not yet able to posit a valid categorisation of discourse types according to their structure; we expect, however, that many information-seeking interviews will have similar structures to the case history section of doctor—patient interviews, and that the interview could well be a discourse type. This linguistic typology might or might not correspond either to lay notions of different situations or to situations of sociological interest.

The claim implicit in the above discussion is that discourse structure is a relatively autonomous level of linguistic organisation which can be studied in its own right — we are *not* making a sociological analysis of doctor—patient interviews, with language data as evidence. Several of the papers in this volume, focusing on processes of construction of everyday life, would deal with the ways people talk as a central feature of that process. From a linguistic point of view, however, they are using the citation and description of isolated speech phenomena as evidence for sociological statements. As outlined in the Introduction, the detailed observation and description of everyday life processes stems from a reaction to the reductionism of previous explanatory theories. However, while reductionism may be avoided by staying close to observed data, there is also a danger that any gain in understanding will be lost if the task of formulating the categories and concepts of more adequate theories is rejected. A non-reductionist explanation and description of social life and language is achieved not by refraining from abstractions, but by taking the longest path from data to explanatory categories; seeing the data as entering into a series of levels of organisation, each partially autonomous but interrelated with other levels. There are tendencies among the school of sociologists calling themselves ethnomethodologists to claim a privileged status for verbal interaction, to treat it as *the* source of social order. For example Dingwall, in this volume, claims that social structures are the outcome of society members' describing and accounting practices and have no existence independent of them. We make no such claim for the level of discourse, but argue only that an adequate understanding of the relation of language and social life must be based on an understanding of the different levels at which language is organised, and that the categories of sociological theories should be related to categories of linguistic description as well as directly to data.

An analogy with sociological treatments of literature may be helpful here. Sociologists have often treated novels as providing a record of social life, from which evidence can be selected for some sociological hypothesis. The character of the novel as a work of art is ignored by this selective approach to literature which wrenches passages from their context. Not only may these passages be misinterpreted, but a richer resource for sociological analysis is wasted. The work of art treated *sui generis* embodies a theory of society that is no longer available to those who attend only to elements of the novel. This point is argued at length in Meyersohn (1969). As Raymond Williams argues, 'This in no way means that the documents are autonomous. It is simply that the significance of an activity must be sought in terms of the whole organisation: which is more than the sum of its separate parts' (Williams, 1965, p. 65).

Our claim then is that, just as literature is a richer source of information about culture and society when its own intrinsic organisation is recognised, so too will sociological studies of language benefit from understanding how language activity is structured in its own right. Sociological categories should not be used to classify stretches of speech as though they had no other organisation: a vast literature exists, particularly on classroom interaction, which raises common sense glosses on types of verbal behaviour to the status of categories for describing stretches of speech (Simar and Boyer, 1968). In this work, as in that by Bales (1951), utterances are categorised directly as providing evidence of the speaker's social role, rather than being first examined to see how they contribute to the ongoing discourse, after which it is possible to see how speakers differ in the characteristic contributions they make to the discourse. The fulfilment of this fiat, of course, depends on linguists providing a model of linguistic organisation that treats language as social behaviour. While linguistics confined itself to the analysis of the phonological substance and the grammatical form of language and treated all else as free variation, all that could be attempted was a correlation between sociological and grammatical categories. Bernstein, the sociologist who above all regarded linguistic organisation as highly important, related his sociological categories to the only available linguistic categories, grammatical ones, and has recently been criticised by Rosen (1972) because the linguistic categories were inadequate.

Our research at the moment concentrates on developing the description of the new linguistic level of discourse which mediates between sociological and grammatical categories. However, the description of discourse structure is one task, the understanding of its interrelations with both grammar and social life another. Because of disciplinary boundaries our competence is in dealing with discourse and grammar and we are concentrating on discovering and describing how participants produce and interpret coherent discourse according to general rules and structures — our ideas on the links between discourse and social life may prove inadequate.

The results of the earlier stage of our work, on classroom discourse, are described in Sinclair and Coulthard (1974). Because we assume that there is linguistic as well as social organisation in verbal interaction, we expect the organisation of discourse to be of the same general type as that at other linguistic levels. Our analysis of discourse structure has proceeded largely by analogy from syntax and phonology.

Briefly, we were able to show that lessons have a fairly complex linguistic structure. Just as the grammatical unit *sentence* can be shown to be composed of one or more *clauses*, which are composed of one or more *groups* or *phrases*, composed of one or more *words* composed of one or more *morphemes*, so we were able to describe a hierarchy of discourse units also in a 'composed of' relationship — *lesson, transaction, sequence, exchange, move, act.*

At present we are not in a position to offer a theoretical justification for this model of discourse structure rather than another; in fact, we expect to find it inadequate, since if discourse is a level distinct from grammar it must exhibit some distinctively different patterning; but in its present form it is a fairly simple, certainly practical, descriptive tool.

We have chosen not to present here the entire model of analysis in a systematic fashion since that would take too long and demand a specialised knowledge of linguistics. Instead we intend to outline some of the basic categories of a linguistic model of discourse, and to characterise some of the typical linguistic units through which doctor—patient communication is realised.

## Linguistic Description

The description of doctor—patient interviews presented here is based on twenty-four tape-recorded interviews, nineteen between general practitioner and patient in the surgery, and five first interviews between consultant and patient in a hospital out-patients department. We explained our research interests to the doctors in fairly general terms and left them to approach their patients for permission to record — most of the doctors discussed the matter before the interview, but one or two told the patients afterwards that they had made a recording for research purposes and asked their permission to retain and use it.

We were not present at any of the interviews ourselves because we wanted the interview to be as 'normal' as possible. We realise, of course, that introducing a tape recorder does have some effect, but our experience in a variety of situations shows that people very quickly forget the tape recorder. Even before they forget, the kind of linguistic adjustments they make are, for our purposes, trivial — they may 'put on an accent' or 'speak more grammatically', but the kind of patterning we are interested in is too basic and deep-seated to be altered. Thus, provided we do not place too much reliance on the first few utterances, we feel fairly confident that our tapes are representative.

We discussed the tapes with the doctors afterwards, though not, like Webb and Stimson (see chapter 7), with the patients. One consultant has been particularly helpful and has talked us through his own and some of his colleagues' tapes.

We have so far treated consultant and GP interviews as if they were variants of the same discourse type. Although there are many similarities, this may turn out to have been a misguided decision because there are also some major differences. The most notable derive from the fact that interviews with consultants are very much longer and devoted entirely to case-history taking, while GP interviews are much shorter but have two major stages, a brief history and a prescription.

### Exchanges

The basic unit of all verbal interaction is the exchange. It consists minimally of two successive utterances — one speaker says something and a second says something in return. Anything less than this is not interactive. The exchange is the building block of interaction and all interaction consists of at least one exchange. Interaction on a chance meeting may consist of a single exchange:

*A*   Hi there.
*B*   Hello.

but is much more likely to continue with a series of related exchanges:

*A*   Haven't seen you for a long time, how are you?
*B*   I'm fine — how are you?

We call the utterances that combine to form exchanges *moves*, and speakers produce one or sometimes two moves each time they have a turn to speak. In the constructed example above B's second turn consists of two moves, an answer to A's question followed by a question for A to answer. The first move in any exchange we call *initiating* — it links forward, and places constraints on what can happen next and sometimes on which person should speak. Some initiating moves define a *responding* move as an appropriate next move after the initiation. Responding moves link backwards but make no requirements on what the next move will be or who will make it. Thus, while a speaker who has made an initiating move must give up the floor, one who has made a responding move need not; he can begin a new exchange with an initiating move of his own.

EXCHANGE I
*A* [initiating move]:          What's the time?
*B* [responding move]:     Five twenty-five.
EXCHANGE II
*B* [initiating move]:          Why do you want to know?
*A* [responding move]:     I'm meeting John at quarter-to.

The third type of move that can occur in an exchange we call a *follow-up*. Like the responding move it links back to the previous move, but unlike the responding move it is not required. Follow-up moves comment on, or indicate understanding or acceptance of, what has gone before in the exchange; they follow responding moves and also some initiating moves that do not require a response. They consist of repetitions or rephrasings of what the previous speaker has said or are versions of 'yes'. Both speakers can contribute a follow-up move in any one exchange, but usually only one occurs.

EXCHANGE I
*Doctor* [initiating move]:    You've only had one in all?
*Patient* [responding move]:  Well as far as I know. There's not
                                 been one this severe like.
*Doctor* [follow-up move]:    Yeah.              [Text C2][2]

There are three kinds of exchange that occur in all types of discourse but are specially appropriate to different stages of a doctor—patient interview: *eliciting*, as in the example above, where the initiation is some kind of question and the response an answer; *directing*, where the initiation is some kind of command or instruction: 'open your mouth, Catherine' (GP10); 'could you lift your leg up' (GP15), to which the appropriate response is the requested action; and *informing*, where the initiation is the transmission of some information, as during the prescribing stage: 'it could well be a cyst there, a small cyst, and the treatment for that . . .' for which the appropriate response is an acknowledgement of understanding, 'yes' (GP17).

Moves, and the acts that make up moves, do not correspond directly with grammatical units. A move for instance might be a sentence or a clause or just one word. Nor do the three types of initiating moves correspond with the grammatical distinctions between declarative, interrogative and imperative sentences. A directing move, for example, might be realised by any of these: 'I'd like you to take your shoes off'; 'Could you take your shoes off'; 'Take your shoes off'. Moves and acts are functional, not grammatical, categories. Different moves and acts are defined on the basis of being meaningfully different selections at certain positions in the structure of discourse. While grammatically different sentences may realise one move, identical sentences may have different meanings in discourse depending on where they occur. This structural definition of moves and acts differentiates them from the probably infinite list of speech acts one could compile by thinking of such activities as promising, threatening, suggesting, warning and so on. Labelling utterances with terms like these would produce some kind of functional description of interaction, but would not reveal discourse structure. There is a more detailed discussion of the principles governing the construction of discourse categories and the relation of discourse categories to grammar in Sinclair and Coulthard (1974).

### Initiating and responding roles

A large part of the interview between the general practitioner and his patient and the whole of the case-history-taking interviews between consultant and patient consist of the doctor eliciting information from the patient on his problem and background. The development of the discourse is tightly controlled by the doctor, who decides whether and when the patient shall transmit that information. We noted above that the role of initiator can change after every exchange — the person who responds can begin the next exchange; in fact, the doctor does virtually all the initiating and the patient virtually all the responding. The recurrent types of exchange are doctor-initiated eliciting exchanges rather than patient-initiated informing exchanges.

If a patient does attempt to initiate the doctor doesn't feel he has to respond, in fact he usually avoids responding, and attempts to regain the initiative. In the following example the doctor treats the first initiation as if it were informing, not eliciting, and provides a typical follow-up move; he ignores the second initiation altogether and produces his own.

| | |
|---|---|
| *Patient* [initiation]: | Now then doctor erm could it be anything to do with erm constipation and kidney trouble? |
| *Doctor* [follow-up]: | I see. |
| *Patient* [initiation]: | Would that make me . . . cold kidney trouble er? |
| *Doctor* [initiation]: | Have you been worried about having kidney trouble? |

[Text C4]

The patient's main and sometimes only chance to present the facts as they seem to him occurs at the beginning of the interview when the doctor usually, as recommended in clinical textbooks, offers him the floor with an open question.

What's the main thing that's troubling you at the moment?

[Text C4]

What's been the matter, recently?

[Text C2]

What's your trouble?

[Text GP9]

How are you today?

[Text GP10]

This opening allows the patient the chance to give a fairly lengthy exposition of his problem if he so desires, but only two of our twenty-four patients take this opportunity; all the others provide very short answers and wait for the doctor to question them again. By contrast one can notice that in television discussions utterances between one and two minutes in length typically follow a question, with participants moving from responding to initiating roles. Patients, however, tend to offer a minimal answer and then return the floor to the doctor. Thus, from the very beginning of the interview, the doctor is typically in the initiating and the patient in the responding role. This means that, if at a later stage in the interview the patient has potentially relevant information, he must tie it, or even drag it, into his answer to one of the doctor's questions.

| | |
|---|---|
| *Doctor:* | What's your appetite like? |
| *Patient:* | Well very good I would say . . . er . . . I'm frightened to eat as you might say doctor for fear I'm going to be in trouble with my er constipation sort of business. |

[Text C4]

The doctor, of course, has his own ideas of what is relevant and irrelevant and will interrupt a patient who is wandering. In the following, unique, example a patient does fight for the right to add what she considers relevant information, but eventually yields.

*Doctor:*    When you say suddenly do you mean over a period of er a few minutes or a few hours or a few days or weeks or what?

*Patient:*    Well sort of suddenly I started getting the headaches whereas before I never had any headaches before.

*Doctor:*    Yes, what do you think yourself brought them on?

*Patient:*    erm COULD I CONTINUE? erm a few weeks ago I

*Doctor:*    mm

*Patient:*    started getting some pains here (untranscribable).

*Doctor:*    YES MRS A LET'S JUST TAKE ONE OF THE SYMPTOMS AT A TIME NOW. . . .

[Text C5]

Thus we see that the structure of the interview is not such that the patient describes in detail pains, sensations, happenings which he thinks constitute an illness while the doctor listens and attempts to identify from the lay description the symptoms of one or more medical problems. Instead, the doctor actively seeks the relevant information in a structured way.

The differentiation between doctor and patient in terms of initiating and responding roles can thus be seen to be relevant to sociological concerns with lay and medical conceptions of illness. Medical conceptions are maintained by the doctor in his communication with the patient by being used to structure the patient's very articulation of his own conception of his illness.

### Informant and recipient roles

As we said above, eliciting exchanges consist minimally of two moves, a question and an answer, but often there is a third, follow-up move commenting in some way on the answer. There are basically two kinds of eliciting question, termed in linguistics *wh* and *polar*. *Wh* questions, beginning with words like 'when', 'where', 'why', 'how', 'who', are seeking information; *polar* questions are looking for the answers 'yes' or 'no'. Thus:

*Doctor:*    How long have you had those for?

*Patient:*    Well, I had'm a week last Wednesday.

[Text C2]

*Doctor:*    Do you find that you ever get headaches when you're wearing your glasses?

*Patient:*    Oh yeah I do.

[Text C5]

The commonsense view of the function of a question is that a person who doesn't know the answer is attempting to discover it from someone who does, but this is certainly not always the case. For instance, in the classroom teachers typically ask questions to which they do know the answers in order to discover whether the pupils also know the answer. In this kind of exchange the information in fact passes from questioner to answerer, not from answerer to questioner, and the information is transferred in the third, follow-up, move. Thus:

*Teacher:*    About how long ago was that?

*Pupil:*    Five thousand years.

*Teacher:*    Five thousand years. Yes.

[Classroom text D]

This follow-up move may be recognised by particular lexical items, e.g. 'good', 'that's right', but more often it is only marked by the selection of *high key*, a paralinguistic feature which for present purposes we can characterise as high pitch at the beginning of the utterance.

We call these exchanges *testing* exchanges, and while they are most typical of classroom interaction they do occur in doctor—patient interviews. In the following example the doctor uses a testing exchange to convince a patient that her hypothesis was wrong. The high key 'yes' in the follow-up move, means 'I knew you were going to say "yes", and "yes" is the right answer.'

*Doctor:*    Do you find that you ever get headaches when you're wearing your glasses?

*Patient:*    Oh yeah I do.

*Doctor:*    Yes [the intonation falls sharply from high to low]. So its not true to say its simply when you take your glasses off that you get a headache.

[Text C5]

More usually, of course, in doctor—patient interviews the information is passing from the responding patient to the eliciting doctor. We call these *transfer* exchanges. They sometimes have a third, follow-up, move which in transcript may look identical to the follow-up move in a testing exchange. Thus it may consist of 'yes', or a repetition of what the patient has said, but the words are marked by the paralinguistic feature of *mid-key* not *high key*. The function of this follow-up is to indicate that the doctor is listening and accepting the information provided by the patient:

*Doctor:*    How long have you had those for?
*Patient:*    Well I had'm a week last Wednesday.
*Doctor:*    A week last Wednesday.
         What were you doing at the time?

                                    [Text C2]

There is a third kind of exchange, which we call matching, in which the first speaker presents something for confirmation and the second confirms it. In other words, the assumptions behind this exchange are that both speakers agree about the answer. Matching exchanges are obviously very important in conversations between people who don't know each other particularly well; they enable participants to check whether their ideas, feelings, impressions are similar, and also whether they are interpreting what the other has said correctly. Typically, in doctor—patient interviews a transfer exchange is followed by one or several matching exchanges:

[transfer] ⎧ *Doctor:*  Have you ever had any serious illnesses in the
          ⎨          past?
          ⎩ *Patient:*  No.
[matching] ⎧ *Doctor:*  No rheumatic fever.
          ⎨ *Patient:*  No, doctor.
[matching] ⎧ *Doctor:*  Pleurisy.
          ⎨ *Patient:*  No, doctor.
[matching] ⎧ *Doctor:*  Pneumonia.
          ⎨ *Patient:*  No doctor.

                                    [Text C4]

What the doctor is doing is to spell out some of the conclusions he has drawn from the patient's reply to his original transfer question. If his question meant the same thing to her that it meant to him all these subsequent questions should be unnecessary, but with a new patient the doctor can't be sure.

*Convergence and divergence*

If the doctor accepts the patient's answers in transfer exchanges and the patient agrees with the doctor's hypotheses in matching exchanges, this is one piece of evidence that there is convergence between doctor and patient. This is not always the pattern however. The degree to which the doctor structures the information he elicits from the patient can lead to two problems of which patients frequently complain. Firstly, he may miss one or more symptoms altogether, and thus produce the wrong diagnosis. Secondly, because for him symptoms can be grouped exclusively — for example a patient has either 'pain' or 'discomfort' — he may ask patients who don't fully understand the intended distinction to categorise a sensation as one or the other.

*Doctor:*   But you don't actually get PAIN in the shoulder.
*Patient:*   No . . . a pain . . . something that seems to er . . .
*Doctor:*   You find it difficult to describe.
*Patient:*   Yes doctor.
*Doctor:*   It's not a true PAIN the shoulder . . .
*Patient:*   No . . . not a . . .
*Doctor:*   . . . but a DISCOMFORT.
*Patient:*   It opens and shuts sort of business.
*Doctor:*   Yes yes. Would you describe it as a DISCOMFORT in your shoulder?
*Patient:*   Yes Doctor.
*Doctor:*   Rather than a true PAIN.
*Patient:*   Yes.

[Text C4]

Also, patients may use informally a word that is a technical term for the doctor — thus, one major type of headache is the tension headache. The patient in the following extracts has been complaining of headaches.

*Doctor:*   What what do you feel round here, this is something new, what do you feel around here in the temples?
*Patient:*   Sort of tension.

A short time later the doctor is asserting . . .

*Doctor:*   Now you brought up this question of tension yourself, er, you said that tension tends to bring on pain over the temples.
*Patient:*   Yes, just here.

. . . even though in between the patient has tried to argue that she didn't say that.

*Doctor:*  But have you noticed that if you're under pressure or worried about anything, er, that this tends to bring on a headache?
*Patient:*  Yes, sometimes even if I don't work hard I still, er, you know, get the headache.

[Text C5]

A continual problem for doctors is that patients sometimes diagnose their illnesses before they arrive and may then present facts to support this diagnosis. In the following extract we see the doctor initially refusing and the patient insisting on the fact that his pains are connected with heart trouble.

*Doctor:*  And what's been the matter, recently?
*Patient:*  Well I've er pains around the HEART.
*Doctor:*  Pains in your CHEST then.
*Patient:*  Yeah round the HEART.
*Doctor:*  Whereabouts in your CHEST?
*Patient:*  On the HEART side.
*Doctor:*  Yes.

[Text C2]

What a doctor regards as a heart attack may not be seen as such by a patient; patients have differing views on what constitutes serious illnesses; patients' memories are short. Thus there are passages in transcripts, when doctors appear to be inattentive or completely disbelieving, which can be explained as attempts to ensure that the patient hasn't forgotten something. Here doctor and patient indicate grammatically that they refuse the other's formulation of the problem.

*Doctor:*  How many ATTACKS have you had?
*Patient:*  It's the FIRST ONE.
*Doctor:*  You've only had ONE in all.
*Patient:*  Well as far as I know there's not been one this severe like.
*Doctor:*  Yeah and when do you get THESE . . .
*Patient:*  IT come on very suddenly last Wednesday.

[Text C2]

These differences in vocabulary and grammar indicate the

distance between doctor and patient; they are formulating the problem differently. When they come to agree, either because the doctor accepts the patient's version or the patient produces new facts to support the doctor's suspicion, there is agreement in vocabulary and grammar.

## Sequences

In an ideal world of perfect shared understandings the doctor could ask a question about the patient's problem and the patient would know exactly what information the doctor required him to provide. The business of exchanging information could be accomplished quickly and efficiently within an exchange. Real interaction is rarely conducted with such little trouble. One exchange grows into a sequence of exchanges concerned with remedying misunderstanding and inexplicitness, with checking understanding and adding afterthoughts. The negotiation of a shared orientation between the doctor and patient takes place through the series of exchanges in a sequence, until the doctor is finally able to match a medical diagnosis with the patient's problem.

In some kinds of discourse exchanges are independent of each other and could be shuffled round without making nonsense of the discourse. This is often the case in classroom discourse where the teacher asks a series of separate information questions:

EXCHANGE I

*Teacher:*   What's that?
*Pupil:*   A nail.
*Teacher:*   A nail, good.

EXCHANGE II

*Teacher:*   What's that?
*Pupil:*   A nut and bolt.
*Teacher:*   A nut and bolt, well done.

[Classroom text G]

In this discourse there is close organisation at the level of exchange but no developing topic, and therefore no important sequential structuring. This is also the case where the doctor is asking a ritual series of questions as in the section dealing with the case-history. Unless one of the patient's answers needs explaining, the questions are produced according to a standard list. The order of exchanges is not responsive to ongoing interaction but is predetermined. Here then we have an exception to the general principle that discourse has an emergent structure, created by the interaction of participants at each point in time.

| | |
|---|---|
| *Doctor:* | Bowels are all right. |
| *Patient:* | Yeah. |
| *Doctor:* | Not passed blood in your motions. |
| *Patient:* | No. |
| *Doctor:* | You haven't passed any motions black like tar. |
| *Patient:* | No. |
| *Doctor:* | No blood in your water, no burning when you pass water. |
| *Patient:* | No. |

[Text C5]

More often, particularly in consultant interviews, the doctor makes a series of linked initiations, where subsequent questions are designed to check on understanding or probe further into the patient's answer. We have already mentioned the use of the matching type of proposing exchange here. The doctor can however choose to return the patient's answer to him for remedy without himself offering an interpretation. This can be done in a number of ways. The doctor can simply repeat some item in the patient's answer, marked by high key so the patient is required to elaborate:

| | |
|---|---|
| *Patient:* | I felt a tight pain in the middle of the chest. |
| *Doctor:* | Tight pain [high key, pitch falling from high to low]. |
| *Patient:* | You know like a sort of ache tightness you might say. |
| *Doctor:* | Yeah. |

[Text C2]

Or he can use particular types of meta-questions which again repeat some item in the answer:

| | |
|---|---|
| *Doctor:* | Did they come on gradually or suddenly? |
| *Patient:* | Suddenly. |
| | I'd never had headaches before. |
| *Doctor:* | Mm. |
| | When you say suddenly do you mean over a period of a few minutes or a few hours or a few days or what. |

[Text C5]

Although it would avoid the doctor overstructuring the patient's responses, it has been pointed out through experiments by Garfinkel (1967), that continual use of questions like 'What do you mean' destroys a necessary background assumption of interaction that participants do share some common orientation.

## Larger units

As we said above, the exchange is the basic building block of verbal interaction and exchanges combine to form larger units. It is at this point that our description shows differences between consultant and GP interviews. In consultant interviews exchanges combine to form *sequences*, which in turn combine to form *transactions*; in GP interviews exchanges combine directly to form transactions. Sequences in consultant interviews consist of a series of related exchanges; the first exchange in each sequence is typically a transfer exchange, the other(s) matching exchanges. We have explained above the significance and use of matching exchanges and it is fairly obvious why such sequences should occur in interviews between a consultant and a patient he doesn't know but not between a GP and a familiar patient.

The highest analytic unit, the transaction, is a series of sequences or exchanges concerned with a single topic. Typically the GP interviews have two, one concerned with the discovery of the problem, the second with prescribing. Consultant interviews have many more. Transactions occur also in classroom language where each transaction is concerned with a stage in the lesson. It is one of the functions of a teacher to make the structure of the lesson as clear as possible to the pupils, and we discovered that teachers mark quite clearly the boundaries of transactions. They do this by the use of one of five words which we call *markers*: 'right', 'well', 'OK', 'now', 'good'. When these words are used to indicate boundaries, they are strongly stressed, uttered with a falling intonation, and followed by a short pause. Their normal meaning is suppressed — 'right' has no evaluative function, 'now' no time reference — though at other places in the lesson these same words are used in their usual meanings.

Having marked a boundary, teachers often also stand aside from the interaction for a moment to tell the pupils what the next part of the interaction will be about, using what we call a meta-statement:

[marker]:           Now . . .

[meta-statement]:            . . . today, we are going to do three
quizzes . . .

[Classroom text D]

And sometimes at the end of a transaction they tell the children what
the transaction was about:

[meta-statement]:    So what we've just done is given some energy
to this pen.
[marker]:            Right. Now,

[Classroom text H]

Thus teaching transactions tend to have a structure of boundary
marker, followed by statement of what the transaction will be about,
followed by the burden of the transaction, followed by statement of
what the transaction was about, followed by boundary marker. It is
obviously important that this high degree of meta-structuring occurs
in classroom language — it is not as important in other forms of
discourse, and transactions are not as clearly bounded in
doctor—patient interviews, but doctors do use markers. For
example, a consultant ends a long transaction concerned with the
patient's previous illnesses and operations with a marker before
moving on to a transaction concerned with her relatives' illnesses:

[marker]:    Good.
             What about your mother and fam — father: did they
             live to a good ripe old age?

[Text C4]

A GP similarly indicates the end of the history and the beginning of
the prescription:

[marker]:    Well, all right.
             Well, I'm going to give you an ointment. . . .

[Text GP9]

[marker]:    Right.
             I'd like you to gargle frequently . . .

[Text GP10]

Markers fulfil their major function at the end of the prescribing
transaction. The doctor uses them to indicate that the interview is
over, he has said all he wants to say, and wants to move into what
Schegloff and Sacks (1973) call the *closing sequence*.

There is an important difference in the placement of closing sequences in consultant and GP interviews. In both cases the doctor will produce a final marker, but the consultant does not precede this by any specific pre-closing section. The point at which he produces this ending seems to be determined entirely by his decision that he has all the information he wants. He offers no opportunity to the patient to raise further topics because the ending is not indicated in advance. Typically, the marker follows a question exchange that has no specific characteristics as a 'last question' and is followed immediately with a dismissal:

*Doctor:*    Right.
          Well, if you go along with nurse she'll give you a cubicle and I'll come and see you in a little while Mrs A.
*Patient:*   Thank you.                    [Text GP5]

The GP indicates that he's coming to the close of the interview with his prescription. In one interview the patient wants simply to talk to the doctor and is clearly aware that if he allowed the doctor to get on to prescribing he would be cut short.

*Doctor:*    Well.
          There you are. I'm going to give you some of those tablets again.
*Patient:*   Well, I've already got a bottle full.
                                [Text GP6]

At the end of GP interviews following the doctor's frame the patient seems to be expected to end the encounter with a goodbye.

*Doctor:*    Righto.
*Patient:*   Goodbye doctor.
*Doctor:*    Goodbye Mrs M.
                                [Text GP7]

If the patient doesn't do this a longer closing sequence can occur:

*Doctor:*    One, twice a day, these, and the other tablets are two four times a day.
[marker]:  Good.
*Patient:*   Yes, thank you.
*Doctor:*    Right.
          Thank you.
*Patient:*   Thanks very much.

*Doctor:*    Righto.
             Goodbye Mrs E.

[Text GP8]


CONCLUSION

The analysis of openings and closings is, of course, a study in itself
(Schegloff and Sacks, 1973), and the main work of our analysis of
doctor—patient interviews so far has concentrated on the structures
of information-seeking. We have outlined above the way in which
the doctor controls the interview in order to elicit information as and
when he requires it, and how he deals with attempts by patients to
present information he does not require or to request information he
is not willing to give. We have also shown how units larger than a
single exchange are built up and how they are structured both
linguistically and topically.

   We have not focused on questions that interest both medical
sociologists and the medical profession in general, such as what
constitutes a good or successful interview, how rapport is
established between doctor and patient, whether the doctor has
elicited all relevant information from the patient or whether the
patient has understood all the doctor's instructions. Such questions
lie outside our competence. What we have done is to provide a
linguistic tool that can be used to describe different interviews and
provide objective evidence for differences or similarities which may
have medical or sociological implications.


NOTES

1   This research was funded by the Social Science Research Council (SSRC), to
whom we express grateful acknowledgement, as The Structure of Verbal Interaction
in Selected Situations.

2   The reference code to each extract indicates from which of the twenty-four
interviews it comes and whether the interview was conducted by a consultant (C) or a
general practitioner (GP).

# Accounts of
# Medical Work

# 6  Accomplishing Profession[1]
## by Robert Dingwall

The notion of 'profession' is central to any inquiry into the social organisation of health and illness. It is, however, a concept that is notorious for the diversity of ways in which it is defined and used by sociologists. It is my contention that this confusion results from the sociologists' treatment of lay social theories as impoverished sociological theorising rather than as phenomena to be studied in their own terms. In this chapter, I shall attempt to develop such an alternative, drawing on my work on the social organisation of health visitor training.[2]

I begin by briefly reviewing the dominant 'attribute' approach to thinking about profession and the main criticisms of it, which one may broadly identify as structural, political and epistemological. My argument will be that each of these criticisms is, in its own way, inadequate and that we should, rather, proceed to the empirical investigation of members' commonsense knowledge of social structures. We should, therefore, abandon any claim to legislate a 'correct' use of the term 'profession' but treat it as a members' concept and seek to describe its practical usage in everyday life.

### SOCIOLOGISTS AND 'PROFESSIONS'

The attribute approach is based on the assumption that it is possible to draw up a list of fixed criteria for recognising a profession on which there will be a general consensus. These criteria can then be used to distinguish between 'professions' and 'other occupations' in a relatively clear and unproblematic fashion. Becker identifies the origin of this approach as a paper published by Flexner in 1915 which set out six criteria of professional activity as

> . . . basically *intellectual*, carrying with it great personal responsibility, it was *learned*, being based on great knowledge and not merely routine; it was *practical*, rather than academic or theoretic, its *technique* could be taught, this being the basis of professional education; it was strongly *organised* internally: and it was motivated by *altruism*, the professionals viewing themselves as working for some aspect of the good of society. [Becker, 1970, p. 88]

In reviewing this literature, Roth (1974) has catalogued a number of more recent attempts to draw up lists and shows how they are all quite different, although there are some points of overlap. But it is clear that these writers are not altogether happy with their acts of definition. Flexner, for example, qualified his whole analysis by saying that

> What matters most is professional spirit. All activities may be prosecuted in the genuine professional spirit. . . . The unselfish devotion of those who have chosen to give themselves to making the world a fitter place to live in can fill social work with the professional spirit and thus to some extent lift it above all the distinctions which I have been at such pains to make. [Flexner, 1915]

The logical outcome of this attribute approach is that a profession is nothing more or less than what some sociologist says it is. He derives his definition from his own member's knowledge of his society or from an inspection of some collection of data. In either case he is basically legislating a social structure by fiat, which as we shall see lays it open to the same objections as any other form of inquiry by fiat.

There are, however, more conventional critiques of this approach. The classic exposition of the structural alternative is presented by Freidson (1970, 1971). He argues that one can distinguish between adopting an ideology of professionalism, which displays the various kinds of features described by the attribute theorists, and the location 'profession' within a given social structure. The recognition of this status is a licence of functional autonomy, secured from the State by political action, giving the profession the exclusive right to control the access to and organisation of the tasks that constitute its work. But such structural considerations, Freidson argues, only set the broad limits of professional performances. The routine conduct of professionals depends upon the concrete features of their everyday work settings. One can question the empirical adequacy of Freidson's approach. The notion of autonomy is highly specific to American practice. Gill and Horobin (1972) note how this is restricted by state intervention in Britain without affecting the social prestige of the occupation. To invert the argument, health visiting, with its independent access to and control over its work, satisfied Freidson's criteria for a profession. Yet I have no grounds for supposing that it would be generally regarded as such.

The key weakness of Friedson's approach is that he is trying to perform the same kind of operation as the attribute theorists. Just as Flexner thought he had found a fundamental criterion in 'professional spirit', so Friedson believes he has found one in 'professional autonomy'. There is a central ambiguity in his work between specifying an *objective* definition of 'profession' and examining the *subjective* knowledge of society members. Freidson is not clear whether he wants to study a collectivity by fiat or through an analysis of the work by which its members make it real for one another. The strain is usually resolved in favour of the former.

The second main line of criticism is political. This presents itself in two forms. The 'hard' version, for example in the work of Illich (1973), argues that the notion of profession is a concept that is used solely to achieve the successful mystification of a class interest. Such an approach, however, takes the reality of labels like 'profession' and 'class' for granted, assuming they are identifiable entities that are unproblematically recognisable and that the sociologist has a special, privileged right to legislate their existence. The 'soft' version of this critique is found in the work of Parsons and Becker. Parsons (1954) notes the coexistence, in modern society, of a capitalist economic order with the development of professions and the traditional dichotomy between analysing the motivations of capitalists in terms of self-interest and of professionals in terms of disinterestedness. He argues that their motivations are similar since each is searching for success, but that they are identified by different sets of imputed motives. He attempts to specify the vocabularies that are drawn upon to impute motives to professionals and businessmen, the 'functional attributes'. This attempt has often been criticised, on empirical grounds, as inaccurate; that we more frequently see moral imperialism than affective neutrality and so on. I would argue that the attempt is limited rather than erroneous. The vocabularies identified by Parsons are invoked by some members in bringing off their sense of location within a social structure. The social distribution of motive ascription is an important element of accomplishing a social structure.

The variant on this 'soft' political theme advanced by Becker (1970) derives directly from his epistemological criticism of the use made by sociologists of the concept of profession. He points out that most of the sociologists' difficulties stem from the use of one word to do two different jobs. While laymen use the term to make moral evaluations of occupations, sociologists use it to point to an 'objectively discriminable class of human phenomena'. Becker argues that this attempt should be abandoned and 'profession' treated as a 'folk concept'; as a part of the vocabulary of social analysis available to members of a collectivity. He tries to do this by treating the work of attribute theorists as data revealing commonsense conceptions of professional work, and he concludes by considering the relation between this popular symbol and 'what really happens'. This returns Becker to the problem of reconciling the objective social order laid down by sociologists, the reality, with the subjective order of collectivity members, the symbol. This leaves him open to the criticisms that Zimmerman and Wieder (1971) make of Denzin (1971) concerning, in particular, the interactionists' assumption that a social world exists 'out there'. The achievement of this appearance of social order is treated as a fact rather than a problem.

The central problem with all these attempts to define 'profession' is their assumption that it has a fixed meaning. On the contrary, I would argue, with Wittgenstein (1972), that words do not have fixed meanings and unequivocal uses according to some calculus of rules. Their sense is found by a process of filling in until we can say that we understand. We cannot, then, define what a profession is. All we can do is to elaborate what it appears to mean, to use the word and to list the occasions on which various elaborations are used. Past approaches pretend to some basic, simple *super*-order of *super*-concepts that are prior to members' experience. But that experience 'is in order as it is', however vague or incoherent it may be.

## An Alternative Approach

How can we bring 'profession' back from its metaphysical to its everyday use? Some clues are provided by Moerman's (1974) discussion of the concept of 'tribe' as used by anthropologists and by his native Lue subjects. He notes the difficulties faced by anthropologists when they attempt to legislate ethnicity by fiat and argues that the relevant question to ask is not 'Who are the Lue?' but 'When and how are the Lue?' He presents a list of traits that Lue invoke to identify themselves as distinct from their neighbours. Many of these are 'objectively' shared with this other people but may still be used by Lue to demonstrate their ethnicity. They identify themselves as Lue and then find the meaning of that identification by elaborating an indefinite set of criteria.

Thus, I set out to examine the use of the term 'profession' by health visitors in relation to their own or other people's behaviour in elaborating 'professional' and 'non-professional' conduct. I then tried to see whether members made empirical associations between this term and others in such a way as to constitute a more or less organised sense of social structure. This meant abandoning any attempt to legislate the definition of a 'profession' and instead involved the study of its usage to establish the activities of health visitors as a 'profession' rather than an 'occupation'. However, as the account shows, these tasks are not completely separable. As well as bringing off 'profession', in opposition to 'occupation', health visitors are also accomplishing 'health visitor' as opposed to 'hairdresser' or 'bricklayer'. The result of this analysis was the following formal scheme, which summarises the empirical work. This is discussed in its entirety elsewhere (Dingwall, 1974). The present chapter will confine itself, by way of illustration, to some aspects of the personal qualities of a health visitor and of the relationship between health visitors and other workers.

## The Formal Scheme

A field health visitor is a professional because:
1. She is a certain sort of person, in that:
    1.1 She has certain ambitions and is committed to her occupation.
    1.2 She has certain personal qualities.
    1.3 She dresses in a certain fashion.
    1.4 She carries herself in a certain way.
    1.5 She uses a certain vocabulary of discourse.
    1.6 She uses certain kinds of transport.

2. She has autonomy in her work and knows what is best for her clients. It follows that:

    2.1   No other health visitor will interfere with her clients.

    2.2   No other health visitor will give her orders about her action towards her clients.

    2.3   No other health visitor will give her clients advice that might conflict with hers.

    2.4   She initiates her own contacts.

    2.5   She is self-critical.

    2.6   She enjoys her work and does not require to be stimulated to do it.

    2.6.1   But she does not work to excess at the expense of her own leisure.

3. She is a member of an occupation which:

    3.1   Selects its recruits.

    3.2   Has formal qualifications.

    3.3   Is self-governing.

    3.4   Has its own body of knowledge.

    3.5   Has a history.

    3.6   Has research done on it.

4. She has responsibility for supervising the work of others such as:

    4.1   Clinic attendants.

    4.2   Health assistants.

5. She is equal to all other professionals but has a discrete area of work. Other professionals include:

    5.1   Social workers.

    5.2   Doctors.

    5.3   Teachers.

    5.4   University staff.

    5.5   Nurses.

    5.6   Various therapists.

6. She acts towards others on the assumption that they share this definition of her social location in an empirically identical (for all practical purposes) fashion.

This list should not be regarded as definitive or exhaustive, but it seems to me to represent an adequate summary of the field data. Competent performance appears to involve giving attention to those elements of this list that are relevant for the management of the particular situation under discussion. Hence we should not expect to find all the elements in any one encounter. This summary, however, by collapsing a variety of situations, might plausibly correspond to some more or less organised interpretive scheme held by members of the health visiting community.

## PROFESSIONAL QUALITIES

Certain features are taken to constitute professional conduct in the eyes of the gatekeepers to health visiting, tutors and senior community health staff, and relate to what one might call existential qualities of the individual health visitor. In order to succeed as a student it is centrally important to establish that one is the right sort of person to be a health visitor. Academic ability is not enough. Assessment of a student is an evaluation of the total person as revealed in everyday activities.

The relevant personal qualities may be stated explicitly as, for example, in this extract from a lecture on health visiting practice:

> Some skills and qualities are required for efficient planning. For instance the skill of organisation, of being able to work out a method, of being methodological. . . . There are other qualities [a health visitor] needs such as being able to adapt to a new area, to be flexible, since anything may disrupt her plans, and to have a sense of humour about this, to be realistic, since she's not going to turn the world upside down because she hasn't got the resources. She should be punctual and reliable and not make rash promises. She needs a sense of humour, a balanced mind and the ability to carry on in spite of obstacles.

Other relevant qualities include ambition for success as a health visitor, as measured by occupation of senior posts and involvement in strategic planning and disseminating innovation, commitment to the occupation, confidence in one's abilities and personal maturity. These features were also recognised by students, although they had their own ways of describing them.

> Clare says the attraction of health visiting is that there is no evening or weekend work. One of the others asked her if she'd said that at the interview. Clare laughed and replied 'No. I said with all my qualifications it seemed a waste not to. Big-head!'.

This extract also shows how students have to present themselves differently to tutors and to other students in order to be recognised as reasonable and rational. Personal qualities may also be revealed in discussion of what a professional health visitor is *not*. The following quotations are taken from an examiners' discussion of possible course failures.

Miss Lane says the student's fieldwork assessor described her as 'shy and diffident' but the tutors feel she lacks articulacy. Her fieldwork instructor described her as 'passive . . . absolutely non-communicative'.

The external examiner says that this student has a more plausible manner but her approach is superficial and there is an element of rigidity in doing an analysis of situations. They felt that this student's inflexibility of attitude could be a danger in the community.

The first student failed because she had been unable to produce acceptable displays of professionalism. The second failed because her performances were felt to lack sincerity. This underlines my original point about the existential nature of these qualities. The performance *is* the person. As one tutor phrased it, 'We see her as a professional, a member of the health service team. When we talk of her role we are talking about the kind of person that she is.' This running-together of doing and being characterises the other elements grouped in this section.

Goffman (1971, pp. 28—82; 1972a, pp. 128—30) has described something of the relevance of props as integral parts of the process of laying claim to be a particular sort of person in any particular encounter. The references made by staff to dress and to cars are instances of such usage. At the time of this research, there was some controversy over whether health visitors should wear a uniform. This was linked to changing conceptions of the sort of person a health visitor should present herself as being, and the relationship she should seek to develop with her clients. Uniforms were felt to create social distance and to imply an authoritarian personality. The abolition of uniforms was associated with progressive trends in health visiting. But not all civilian dress was equally acceptable. Trousers were disapproved of for women. Male health visitors felt required to wear jackets on duty, even on hot afternoons in inner London. The clothing credits that the local authority in the City substituted for a uniform could be drawn on only at one of six rather old-fashioned department stores. Similar points can be made in relation to car ownership. The specification of the social meanings of modes of transport is a large topic and I shall confine myself to two examples here. The first is from a verse in circulation in the early sixties quoted by McQueen (1962) and the second is from a local newspaper.

As the HV and the Midwife pedalled fiercely in the rain
The Schoolmarm in her Austin looked upon them with disdain
And the half-trained Welfare Worker ran her mini-car quite well.

A full-page article [in the official magazine of the Police Federation] by a member of the Cheshire force which has decided to retire its Panda cars expresses regret for the backward trend. Apart from the technical advantages, he argues, Pandas raised the job 'almost, if not financially, to the level of a profession'.

Car ownership was a prop in the health visitors' claims to professional status. It was also linked with the switch from district work to practice attachment.

The accomplishment of health visiting as a profession also required the adoption of certain forms of communication, both linguistic and paralinguistic. Schutz (1970, p. 14) observes that,

The vernacular of everyday life is primarily a language of named things and events and any name includes a typification and generalisation referring to the relevance system prevailing in the linguistic in-group which found the named thing significant enough to provide a separate name for it.

One of the problems of demonstrating the identity of health visiting is its lack of such a language. This reflects its interstitial position between the health and welfare services. Its vocabulary is loosely drawn from nursing, medicine and social work. There is, for example, no term to describe the persons in receipt of services. They may be referred to as 'patients', 'clients', 'families', 'mothers', 'people' or 'the ladies I go to visit'. On the other hand, there is only one acceptable way of describing a health visitor and that is as a 'professional'. Since health visitors cannot be identified by a special vocabulary, the emphasis shifts to the form of their communications. Appeals are made to some shared sense of appropriate language. Professionals, should not, for example, use local dialect.

> Alice says it can be very patronising for an outsider to use dialect. Miss Lane says the point is rather different. 'We are going in as professional workers and I do honestly feel we have to be ourselves in that role.' She adds that it is wrong to adopt the clients' language but that you do have to understand it.

This point also received attention in criticisms of their teaching practice and the need to select a style that was neither too technical nor too informal.

In conclusion, we should also note what, following Birdwhistell (1973), we might describe as the kinesic dimension of professional performance. Birdwhistell argues that the management of body shapes and movements is a learned accomplishment which takes place inside a given cultural frame. Just as we can recognise membership of a collectivity through mastery of its natural language, so too we should be able to recognise kinesic communities bounded by learnt systems of body management. The present research did not investigate such phenomena in detail by using some notational system, but it did turn up examples of professionalism being formulated in terms of correct and incorrect body management. Thus, one student recounted how she had been criticised on teaching practice for not looking elegant enough and for leaning on the table while talking. The assessor had said this was 'unprofessional'. Other students had had similar experiences. Tutors drew attention to the problems involved in relating to children at their own level while trying to bring off a professional performance for parents. Davis and Strong, elsewhere in this volume, describe similar difficulties for play therapists. Body management could also be used as a discriminator between health visiting and other occupations and as an area for conflict over definitions of correct performance.

The first three sections of the formal scheme list features of the qualities of performance and of the organisation of health visiting work that contribute towards the health visitors' definition of themselves as professionals. The accomplishment of health visiting as a 'profession' involves its members in *being* certain kinds of people who carry out tasks in particular kinds of ways within a particular work setting. But a claim to professional status involves more than this. It is also the assertion of a claim to a particular kind of social location in relation to other social groups. It is to this claim that I shall now direct my attention.

## PROFESSIONS AND OTHER OCCUPATIONS

Health visitors' claims to professional status are based upon their ideas about the social structure of their society and of the relative placing of occupations within it. This involves the location of the occupation as equal, inferior or superior to others. This self-location may not, of course, be recognised by members of those other occupations, and there is no reason why it should be. The ideas about the structure of a society that members of that society draw on to inform their actions towards other members are necessarily socially distributed. This is because different groups need to draw on different sets of ideas in order to demonstrate that their members are both reasonable and rational. It clearly offers a point of potential conflict and can also raise questions about differential ability to enforce conceptions of social structure. In this chapter I shall concentrate on those groups identified by health visitors as social equals. These included doctors, nurses, social workers, teachers and various types of therapist. Those considered as social inferiors included clinic staff, health assistants and some government services. I found no instances of groups regarded as social superiors.

Occupations may be regarded as the outcome of social schemes of classification of work. The study of occupational systems is the study of taxonomies of social phenomena. We can, then, treat occupational taxonomies as we might any other folk taxonomy, examining the methods whereby categories are formulated, the ways in which phenomena are recognised and assigned and the system as a whole is described and justified. Further, we can consider what is involved in maintaining the taxonomy's orderly character, and the ways in which new cases are normalised by identifying them as instances-of-a-type. The interstitial position of health visiting in the welfare state raises particular difficulties for such processes. It is neither entirely a health service nor entirely a social service. This gives prima facie grounds for expecting to find problems of *exclusion*, of defining oneself as a discrete occupation. But the groups from which health visitors wish to distinguish themselves are also those with which they rank themselves socially. Thus we might find problems of *inclusion* and the question of how health visitors manage to regard such occupations as the same but different. I shall, then, present a number of instances of health visitors talking about other occupations, and shall attempt to make a number of inferences about the kind of social order that is being formulated through that talk.

The relationship that health visitors formulate with respect to doctors raises problems of inclusion, of achieving recognition as social equals. As we have seen, health visitors are encouraged to define themselves as professionals and to act towards doctors on the basis of this self-definition and on the basis of defining the profession of medicine as embracing similar features, and to anticipate the reciprocation of such expectations. On the whole, these expectations are frustrated. I shall, then, begin by considering the models of health visitor—doctor relations held by the respective parties and then examine the ways in which the difficulties arising from the discrepancies between the models are managed.

In their encounters with health visitor students, I identified two doctors' models of their relation with health visitors. The first was held by staff from the local medical school who talked freely about changing relationships between various health workers and the emergence of a team of equals integrating both hospital and community services. They were enthusiastic about the 1974 health service reorganisation. Their conception of the team included the possibility of an independent role for health visitors and, indeed, the possibility that the team might not be led by a doctor. They were sceptical, however, about the extent to which such views were shared throughout their occupation. Most of the general practitioners seemed to work with a second model. These people saw the primary health care team as a group of auxiliary workers who would be organised and directed by the general practitioner. While these auxiliary workers might have skills of their own, they merely duplicated in a rather partial way those of the doctor himself and were to be used strictly under his supervision. He would be responsible for the definition, allocation and pacing of the workloads. The model drawn upon by the health visitors is well summarised in a paper that the tutors circulated to the students.

Each member of the team should understand and respect the roles and functions of every other member of the team. This implies partnership not hierarchy. In particular the nurse members of the team are partners with and not ancillary to the medical members of the team. Nursing is a professional skill in its own right, requiring a specific professional preparation; doctors are not in a position to assess nursing needs nor to supervise nursing practice.

Health visiting had its own area of expertise in which health visitors did better than doctors and for which doctors were not competent supervisors.

When groups, such as general practitioners and health visitors, invoke such radically different models of the proper relation between them, one might expect to find conflict when they actually come face to face in everyday working situations. In the event, however, there was relatively little that I could identify as direct confrontation. The doctors assimilated health visitors into their typification of nurses and the health visitors tended to slip into this model of social relations, while at the same time recognising its discrepancy with their preferred version of events. They relied on traditional nurses' strategies of indirect negotiation like those described by Stein (1968) to press policies on the doctors. Of course they had greater resources for this than nurses since they had independent access to their clientele, and could influence self-referral for treatment by influencing patient demands and tactics. For example, where a health visitor disagrees with a doctor's prescribing policies she can seek to encourage or dissuade patient requests for medication. Similarly, health visitors in one area which I studied coached women seeking abortions in the right ways of beating the local system in which the consultants operated a restrictive policy. Other nurses can only manage information about patients after they have been committed to their care.

Such activities, however, were tempered by the requirement to accomplish profession in respect of the public at large and to maintain the integrity of interprofessional relations to the public. As I suggest in section 2 of the list of qualities involved in accomplishing profession, it is important that the integrity of each professional's independent judgement be maintained. Thus, although health visitors, particularly on district work, have a considerable store of comparative knowledge on the quality of individual general practitioners, they were unable to put this at their clients' disposal. They sought to encourage people to patronise 'good' doctors but could not discourage them from going to 'bad' doctors. In comparing the contraceptive advice given by general practitioners and family planning clinics, for example, they would emphasise the advantages of the clinic, such as free supplies and specialist knowledge, rather than the inadequacies of the general practitioners.

It would seem that health visitors remedy the difficulties generated for them by the discrepancy between their 'ideal' and 'real' models of social structure through their conversations about doctors. The telling of 'atrocity stories' is an important dimension in the constitution of the occupational group, which may be defined in terms of those to whom one tells such stories and from whom one receives them. Thus, although health assistants, clinic attendants and sociologists may on occasion be allowed to listen, it is out of order for them to tell such stories. Story-telling in relation to general practice consultations is discussed elsewhere in this volume by Webb and Stimson. They contend that stories can be seen as devices whereby patients redress the imbalance in the relationship between doctor and patient by allowing the voicing of complaints at a safe distance. The teller is presented as being sensible or rational in the face of the incompetence or dereliction of doctors. The rational nature of the social order is made evident as the patient reconstructs the scene as he would have liked it to have been. I would argue that such story-telling is similarly bounded to people-like-oneself, but that the work that is accomplished is a common feature of everyday life. In the face of the persistent infringements of our sense of our own rationality which are the inevitable outcome of the distribution of ideas about the nature of our society and of the ability to enforce one's own version as essentially correct, stories allow us to reconcile everyday events with our ideals and for our peers to reaffirm our sense of our own rationality.

Health visitors commonly tell stories about doctors, particularly in the presence of students. This would seem to involve two kinds of issues. Firstly, there is the demonstration of the rationality of one's occupation before novices for whom such a proposition might seem questionable. Secondly, there is the transmission of the social theories which the student is likely to need to draw on to mount a competent performance as a health visitor. Over time, the students develop their own repertoire of stories. Initially, they talked about how they had successfully compensated for the deficiencies of doctors in the hospitals in which they had worked. As they accumulated experience in health visiting work, stories about health visitors and doctors appeared, drawing either on the students' own experience or upon accounts transmitted by field staff. Space does not allow me to give illustrations but the stories share the same features as those presented by Stimson and Webb (1975) casting the teller as the active participant who sets things right despite the incompetence and idiocies of others.

The problems posed for health visitors by nursing and social work were rather different, being problems of exclusion. Health visiting was seen as overlapping considerably with the work of each of these groups and this presented difficulties in demarcating health visiting as a separate occupation. Indeed, there were those who would argue at times that health visiting was 'really' social work or nursing. The present account concentrates largely on relations between health visiting and nursing occupations — hospital nursing, midwifery and district nursing — but much of the material relating to social workers is broadly similar.

The issue of distinguishing health visiting from nursing chiefly arose in the early weeks of the course. To some extent, it was deliberately raised by tutors in the context of reformulating student conceptions of everyday life. These conceptions may be thought of as akin to Schutz's (1962) notion of provinces of meaning, with their own peculiar cognitive styles and socially distributed stocks of knowledge. For if we are to regard the reality of everyday life as constituted for collectivity members by their everyday routine actions and the recipes which enable them to produce and recognise such actions, and if knowledge of such recipes is socially distributed, then the sense of the reality of everyday life must itself be socially distributed. But since our social, as opposed to physical or temporal, locations may change infrequently or only gradually it is difficult to make abrupt changes in our commonsense notions of social structures. However, organisations, like schools, which specialise in changing such commonsense notions, develop routine ways of accomplishing the transition. In the school of health visiting, the tactic was to reformulate the students' past to include it within their present. Once this had been done the distinctiveness of the present situation was re-emphasised.

This reformulation partly involves a manipulation of health visiting history to emphasise its association with nursing and its connection with important symbolic figures like Florence Nightingale. The concept of an 'official history' as a legitimation of the present state of affairs by selective attention to historical events is discussed more fully elsewhere (Dingwall, 1974). For the present, suffice it to say that many other possible histories are available but that this is the particular one that occurs. The tutors at the school gave explicit attention to definitional questions, underlining the continuity between health visiting and nursing. Where distinctions were discussed, tutors stressed the positive qualities of health visiting, its particular satisfactions, authority style and training rather than the negative qualities of nursing. However, with the passage of time the staff's remarks to the students became more pointed. They criticised the rigid hierarchical structures of nursing and the authoritarian leadership of senior personnel. Student nurses, they said, were reduced to passivity by this. Their training had low educational standards, was poorly taught and rather uncritical. Patients were reduced to objects of task performance rather than being treated as human beings with their own thoughts and feelings. This legacy from the past, said the staff, hampered their efforts to produce good health visitors. The health visitor students were very unwilling to accept the staff's criticisms of nursing at the beginning of the course, although they recognised them, but as time went on began to give similar accounts themselves. One must not discount the role of selection and self-selection in this, but since the students found such difficulty in constructing a coherent account of health visiting, and since these accounts related to reasons for leaving nursing rather than for becoming a health visitor, I think we may reasonably conclude that this is what nursing is like for some of those experiencing it as an occupation.

ACCOMPLISHING PROFESSION

This account has brought us some way from our original starting point in an attempt to provide a more adequate conceptualisation of the notion of a 'profession'. I readily concede its shortcomings, in particular in relation to its handling of evidence. Space has not permitted the analysis of detailed conversational data. Nevertheless, I have tried to offer an alternative to the legislation of social order involved in previous attempts at the analysis of the term 'profession'. In particular, I have suggested that we need to examine how occupations are distinguished from one another through the interpretive work of their members and of outsiders, and further how certain occupations seek to establish themselves as 'professions' through certain kinds of appeals. We need studies of the appeals that are made by members of an occupation, the ways in which they are made and in what settings they are made in order to accomplish that occupation as a 'profession'. Further, we require details of the response of others to such work. This points the way, for example, to studies of the transmission of social theories through education and communications media and to the use of such theories in everyday situations. The injunction is, ultimately, to take the everyday world of the non-sociologist seriously rather than to substitute our own versions of reality for it.

## NOTES

1 The research discussed in this paper was carried out while in receipt of a Medical Research Council Research Studentship.

2 Health visitors are public health nurses who have received a post-basic training in an institution of tertiary education. They are concerned with preventive health and social advice among particular categories of the population. They have a statutory responsibility for the routine visiting of all mothers and young children, regardless of circumstances, and also work with antenatal women, old people and sufferers from various chronic diseases. Their work has no direct clinical component, being exclusively educative and advisory. On the whole they have a relatively high standing in relation to registered nurses, being equated for salary purposes, for example, with ward sisters.

# 7 People's Accounts of Medical Encounters

## by *Barbara Webb and Gerry Stimson*

As part of a study of the consultation process in general practice (Stimson and Webb, 1975) we collected people's verbal accounts of 'what happened'. We wish, in this chapter, to compare these 'lay' accounts with our own observations of the consultation process. In the accounts that people gave of their consultations the patient is portrayed as having taken a very active part in the encounter, and the patient's opinions, judgements and subjective feelings figure prominently. Our own observations, by contrast, reveal the patients as less directive and less active than the doctor and rarely making their feelings explicit.

We see the person's consultation with the general practitioner as part of an extended process involving the patient-to-be in a whole series of prior anticipations, expectations and preparations for the encounter and, after the consultation is over, involving the person in evaluation and appraisal. It is during this period of reappraisal and evaluation when there may be verbal accounts of 'what really happened'.

Approximately fifty consultations between patients and doctors were observed in a South Wales town. These form the main source of our sociological account of the consultation. For the patient's point of view we draw on material from two sources. First, we conducted group discussions on subjects related to health, illness, doctors and medical care. The participants were all women who knew each other. Second, we recorded accounts of consultations that we overheard, or in which we ourselves were involved, in everyday conversation. This latter source provided us with a wealth of processual material spanning several months concerning a small number of people who, while they were not aware of our record-keeping, were aware of our research interests. These latter accounts were not about the particular consultations that we observed. Because our patient accounts were from women, we have in this chapter confined all our consultation examples to women.

## THE PATIENT'S ACCOUNT

All talk can be used as a source of accounts but we shall emphasise one style of talk — the story — because this figured prominently in our material. We shall not ignore the other talk about doctors which we recorded, but we soon became aware that there were certain typical ways of talking about experiences with the medical profession which we began to call 'atrocity stories', 'critical stories' or 'typical stories'. These accounts were rather vivid descriptions of such things as attempts to see the doctor, hospital experiences, the drugs that doctors had prescribed, home visits by the doctor and consultations in the surgery. We were alerted to the 'story-telling' nature of these accounts partly by the comments that some people made on finishing their account — 'It's a hair-raising story isn't it?' — and partly because of the way these accounts were introduced.

We argue that the story is a form of communication by which people make sense of past events. It is a means of accounting for or explaining the social world of, in this case, doctors and patients. Furthermore, we see the way in which people reconstruct the encounter from their own perspective as deriving from the more passive part they play in the consultation. In telling the story the integrity of the patient is affirmed or maintained.

The story form of recounting has the following characteristics:

(i) The presence of and reaction of an audience. When stories began other conversation ceased. Sometimes stories would be prompted by one person who requested the story from another: 'Tell them about the time you . . .'. It was often obvious that we, as researchers with a tape recorder, provided an ideal audience for the recounting of stories. Sometimes one story would follow another in a complementary or competing fashion.

(ii) That stories are prompted suggests that they have been told before and are now being repeated. This implies that, rather than being simply a way of reporting an event, the audience appreciates the repetition of 'a good story'.

(iii) The stories have a dramatic quality. They begin with the scene being set, the characters introduced, the problem explained. As the plot unfolds the major areas of conflict between the participants are revealed.

(iv) There is a shared understanding of the expressions used, and in the taken-for-granted assumptions that are omitted from the story (Garfinkel, 1964). Statements like 'and I noticed her going downhill', 'I put it down to the smallpox injection', and 'back and fro to the doctors' are assumed by the speaker to be understandable to the audience and therefore do not require elaboration. Large portions of the action may be omitted without the teller having to explain this to the listeners.

(v) The stories are told as eye-witness accounts. Usually they are of experiences that the teller has undergone, or of experiences of close friends or relatives. The stories have a highly personal content and involve the audience by virtue of the teller's ability to portray and the listener's ability to realise that 'this sort of thing has happened to me and might happen to you'. The listeners are thus encouraged to feel sympathy and common understanding with the teller. The characters are portrayed as 'real' people and the incidents 'actually happened'.

For the purpose of our analysis, we do not make any claim about the correspondence between what is depicted in the stories and what 'independent observers' might agree to have happened at the incident in question. Our interest is in the way the stories are told and not in questions of the validity of the accounts. We have dealt with an analysis of the stories in some detail elsewhere (Stimson and Webb, 1975). For the present discussion we are concerned with two features of the stories: the way in which the patient and the doctor are portrayed, and the prominence of the feelings of the patient.

## The Portrayal of the Patient in the Story

In the story of some encounter between the teller/patient and the doctor, the former is usually portrayed as playing a very active role.

This is indicated by such sentences as 'And I said to the doctor . . .' or 'And I told him I wasn't having any of that' or at one remove 'We would not have got my father into hospital only for my daughter turning round and saying, "Look doctor, if you don't get him out of here right away I will go right over your head".'

As we have never been present at an encounter that was later retold as a story, it may be that in the type of incidents that become worthy of telling as a story the patient *did* play a very active part. We suspect, however, that the emphasis on the active part played by the patient in the story owes more to the story being a vehicle for making the patient appear rational and sensible, and for redressing the imbalance between patient and doctor, than it does to the event itself.

In the following extract from a story in which a woman describes her traumatic experiences in childbirth, both the woman patient and her husband are verbally active in expressing their feelings to the medical staff. The woman describes herself as 'screaming' her intention not to have the operation, and the angry husband is depicted as giving the staff 'hell'.

> [I was] crying hysterically. . . . I was screaming that I wasn't ever going down to that operating theatre again. When my husband came, well he was livid. He gave them hell. He said he'd never known anything like it — wouldn't have believed it possible if someone had told him about it. After all I'd been through and they knew about the time I'd had. I said I'd never have another child and I'd never go near that hospital again.

Yet the way in which the teller depicts the patient as having taken an active part in the confrontation with the doctor contrasts again with the patient's lack of action in making any formal complaint. A person who can take the initiative might be expected to be equally active in pursuing a complaint. If someone asks why they did not complain the teller must then make accountable this apparent inaction which seems to contradict the active part played by the patient in the reconstructed event. (Our term 'make accountable' is equivalent to Scott and Lyman's, 1968, use of the term 'account' to mean 'a statement made by a social actor to explain unanticipated or untoward behaviour'.) If the story depicts outrageous behaviour on the part of the doctor the teller may appear 'stupid' if nothing was done about it afterwards. In the following transcription, from a group discussion, the teller makes the doctor appear to have acted so irresponsibly that a 'rational' patient would have complained.

*Teller:* I lost my first baby, you see. I had toxaemia, and all the time, you know what you are when it's your first, I didn't go to the clinic, I went to my doctor's antenatal. Well, when I was seven months, I was booked for, he booked me in for a bed in hospital and all that, you know. I went down to the hospital, I was rushed in immediately! My blood pressure was abnormal. I had, oh, I didn't know my doctor had to take my blood pressure. He hadn't been taking my blood pressure. Well the baby died then, it was only two pound born, I had toxaemia which stops the growth or something of the baby and my doctor didn't even take my blood pressure, and I know that, for all those seven months that I had been going to him. I didn't know he had to take my blood pressure you see. But I went down to see. You automatically, if you're booked for hospital, you get a letter to go and see the specialist too, you know, and my blood pressure was abnormal. I was taken in immediately for complete rest.

*Author:* Did you take it up with him afterwards, I mean have you ever complained directly to your doctor?

*Teller:* Oh yes, but he was fantastic to me then when I was pregnant on Stephen you see. He was marvellous. He did, same happened to her [nodding towards friend], he done everything he could do possible then. He looked after me well . . . He couldn't do enough for me then.

This counter-balancing of the atrocity story with a compliment is a face-saving technique which serves to maintain the 'good sense' of the teller. The fact that the doctor was to 'redeem' himself at the time of the second pregnancy could not have been known to the patient at the time of the crisis incident, yet this logical problem was not raised by anyone listening.

As we have seen above, many of the accounts are critical of doctors. Sometimes this comes across as the patient overtly disagreeing with or criticising the doctor, at other times the conflict is implicit in the style of telling which gives the audience the impression that this disagreement was made obvious to the doctor at the time. Story-telling allows grievances to be aired. Equally, it enables these incidents to be related whenever the opportunity arises and allows the values that they affirm to be reinforced. Social reality can be constructed from a safe distance where those on the 'other side' do not have to be taken into account and they cannot themselves dispute that construction.

OBSERVATIONS OF THE CONSULTATION: THE PERFORMANCE OF THE PATIENT AND THE DOCTOR

Before showing how the doctor is portrayed in the patients' stories we now give a brief summary of some of our own observations of consultations. Mauksch (1972) makes a point about the symbolic self-presentation of physicians and nurses in the hospital which is relevant to patient—doctor contacts as these are described by patients:

> Anyone, who had heard physicians talk about nurses in their own lounge, then heard nurses speak among themselves about the medical staff, could never extrapolate from these experiences the language, the behaviour and the relationships which occur as stage behaviour when physicians and nurses meet on the patient care unit, in the conference room or in administrative sessions.

Similarly, we would find it hard to extrapolate from people's stories to the performance of doctors and patients when they meet in the consultation. Our observations of consultations suggest first that patients are much less active and directive in the interaction than the doctor, and less active than they are depicted in the stories, and second that any conflict between doctor and patient tends to be masked, particularly on the patient's side, by a facade of compliance and acquiescence, and that where the patient disagrees with the doctor, and would wish to query or contradict him, then the strategies that are used are covert.

*Presenting a problem to the doctor*

The patient tends not to make categoric statements when talking to the doctor. The patient may have definite ideas about what the symptoms are related to, what they might indicate and the sort of treatment that is appropriate, but when explaining the symptoms to the doctor these ideas are offered only as tentative suggestions:

> I've had a lot of headaches lately — I wondered if it could be anything to do with my blood pressure?

If the patient feels that the doctor is missing the point and needs to be put 'on the right lines' the persuasion is subtle. The doctor's diagnosis is rarely contradicted, but the patient may persist in offering or reiterating what are seen as the salient features of the problem. One young woman, consulting the doctor about her child whose problem the doctor had interpreted as being 'nothing to worry about', reiterated that the child's symptoms were both unusual and worrying.

> Yes, but it's most unusual for him to keep vomiting up his feed like this. And as I say, he's never been like this before.

She rephrased these sentiments three times during the discussion over the child's problem. Coulthard and Ashby analyse similar exchanges in chapter 5.

### Requesting action from the doctor

The patient's request is usually indirect and oblique. In the following example a woman patient tries to persuade the doctor that her problem merits medical attention. She presents her symptoms but the doctor can find no explanation for them in the examination he makes or from the medical history on the patient's record card. The situation appears to be one of stalemate until the patient herself eventually proposes a course of action. She persists in showing the symptoms as a matter of concern and succeeds, by offering a solution of her own, in gaining the doctor's recognition that some action should be taken. The consultation began with the woman describing 'odd pains' and giddiness and complaining that she had put on weight. We begin the dialogue with her speaking while the doctor examines her.

*Patient:*    I've taken tablets, I thought I could fight it off.
*Doctor:*    Mmm. Uh-huh.
*Patient:*    This morning I couldn't even drink my cup of tea so I knew something was wrong.
              [examination ends]
*Doctor:*    Well that's normal, there's nothing wrong there.

*Patient:*   Well I don't know what causes it, I'm sure.
*Doctor:*   Your blood pressure's all right, there's nothing the matter there.
*Patient:*   Nothing to worry about? Oh well, there you are then.
*Doctor:*   Are you sure you've put on half a stone?
*Patient:*   Definitely.
          [Pause in dialogue]
*Patient:*   Is there something I could stop eating? I can't wear my clothes now.
*Doctor:*   Cut out sugar in your tea and flour products, take them only in moderation. Try that and see how you go on. It'll take some time, mind.
*Patient:*   [*laughs*] Oh, I know that!

Both begin to joke about eating and weight problems.


### Questioning the doctor's actions

Patients rarely queried a doctor's past or present performance to his face. Questions to the doctor were phrased in a way that related to the specific problem being presented, and statements were not made that implied general criticism of the doctor's behaviour.

When the patient does ask questions reference is made to the doctor as a representative of medical knowledge rather than asking what the doctor himself can do. The questions are asked in the form 'What can be done?' or 'Is there anything that can be done?' rather than in the personal form of 'What can you do?'

Few patients address their doctor in the manner in which he speaks to them. Of course, patients sometimes make more demanding statements which are direct in form and tone: 'Can't anything be done for it then?' or 'Can I have a sick note for work?' but these are usually of an inquiring nature rather than instructive or evaluative. Consider, in contrast, the judgemental or directive language of the doctor in the following extract from a surgery consultation in which he is commiserating with a woman patient over the behaviour of a 'difficult' daughter:

> She's just stupid . . . she buzzes off whenever she feels like it . . .
> she doesn't want to take responsibility . . . That's what I don't
> understand why she doesn't get a job.

Speech volume also reflects these differences. The patient's speech is generally much quieter than the doctor's, although the volume often increases as the consultation progresses. It may also be used to cover feelings that the patient is unable or unwilling to put into words — patients may mask feelings of disagreement or dissatisfaction behind muttered or mumbled comments that are barely audible.

In general, then, the overt behaviour of the patient tends to be passive compared with the doctor's. The initiative is usually taken by the doctor in pulling the various strands of conversation together and summarising what he considers to be the significant points from the information given by the patient. The doctor defines the significant and will ignore what he sees as irrelevant. This, verbally, is his 'acting like a doctor'. The doctor's directness is most obvious in his ability to control the timing of activities in the consultation. He provides entry and exit cues for the patient — although the patient does have ways of 'stalling for time' or 'hurrying along' the doctor — and in general controls the course of the dialogue. He may interrupt and change the subject. Often these changes are marked or accompanied by non-verbal cues, such as the doctor diverting his attention elsewhere, rising from his chair, picking up or laying down his pen. It is because the doctor regularly and routinely holds consultations that he develops a routine and a range of strategies that he may call upon in his interaction with the patient. The patient is not usually as experienced in 'managing' the consultation or in 'managing' doctors. A doctor at one of the practices that we studied spoke of his methods for getting patients to leave his consulting room:

> Well, after a reasonable period has elapsed and you've achieved what you set out to, there are some who tend to gabble on! — and one or two who don't go, you've got to go through a long formal farewell to get them out. But usually if you simply get up, they do too! And you lead them to the door and before they know it, they're outside.

In view of the way in which the patient behaves, it is not surprising that we rarely observed open conflict or disagreement in the consultation. Furthermore, while the feelings of the patient are prominent in the story, in general the emotional element in the consultation tends to be 'played down' by both doctor and patient, so there is almost an emotional flatness to the consultation. Fears are rarely brought out into the open. However, as we have seen, the lack of drama and emotional expression in the consultation is in marked contrast to the dramatic and emotional content of patients' accounts of their surgery encounters when talking to family and friends (or interviewers).

There also appears to be considerable complicity in the consultation; what in lay terms can be described as 'good manners'. Overt expression of conflict is as rare as the expression of emotion. A patient seldom makes accusations to a general practitioner's face about what are considered to be inefficiencies and inadequacies. Similarly, a doctor rarely loses his temper with a patient. If it appears that this point is being approached, the other actor seems to step down and attempts to avoid the issue or heal the breach. A patient who failed to keep her hospital appointment evoked the doctor's annoyance. During the consultation he said to her:

> Well I'm sorry Betty. What do you expect me to do? I've done as much as I can . . . What's the use if you don't do anything I say?

Betty remained silent throughout, muttering her apologies just before leaving.

The thoughts of the patient that are not articulated during tense or difficult exchanges such as those above may form the basis for stories told about doctors when the patient is well away from the surgery.

## REDRESSING THE INEQUALITIES BETWEEN THE CLIENT AND THE PROFESSIONAL

All our stories were collected from women, and sexual antagonism may be a factor contributing to the emphasis on conflict in the contact between patient and doctor — all the women spoke of male doctors. There is the further possibility that the cultural and class element in the stories is greater than we have supposed; cultural in that the opinions and the way they are expressed reflect some 'Welshness' in our informants, and class in that most of our informants were lower-middle or working class. While there may be such factors that operate to produce different types of contacts between doctors and patients, and different ways of talking about such contacts, we would hold that the experience of being a patient — one aspect of which is the conflict emphasised in these stories — transcends the class and cultural differences that affect the type of contact and relations between particular patients and doctors.

Our observations of the consultation are in marked contrast to people's accounts of what goes on. Why should this be so? It may be that our observations were conducted at surgeries where patients experienced little conflict with the doctors, or that we were not there when it occurred. It may be that our group discussions were held among people who expected us to hear their grievances, or it may be that the critical account makes a 'better story'. Certainly the 'atrocity' story had the greatest dramatic impact on the audience. Despite this, a person who tells a story in which she is highly critical of doctors may then relate an incident in which she has 'nothing but praise' for doctors. The sentiments thus expressed in any one story do not necessarily reflect a general attitude towards the medical profession, but rather reflect some of the inequalities in the relations between doctors and patients.

We have touched on some of these inequalities between the doctor who makes decisions relating to the patient, and who is usually the initiator of action and the principal actor in the encounter between the two, and the patient, who is more passive, and who reacts and responds to the doctor's initiative. The relationship between the professional who dispenses his services and the client who requires some action to be taken by a professional on his behalf is necessarily unequal because it gives control and influence to the professional.

It is difficult in the consulting situation for the patient to show the doctor that she is capable of forming her own opinions and making her own decisions. A patient may ask the doctor's advice, but she rarely tells him if she disagrees with it or has no intention of following it. It is perhaps easier for the patient to remain silent when she has doubts or queries about the doctor's words and actions and can make her own decisions away from the surgery, rather than voice them in the consultation. When the doctor dismisses a problem as unimportant or ignores a symptom presented by the patient, the patient's lack of persistence may not necessarily indicate that she too now perceives that problem as insignificant. It is noticeable in many consultations that, just as the dialogue is drawing to a close, the patient makes frequent agreeing sounds as though these are as appropriate as the farewells and thanks that mark the exit. This formal acquiescence, however, is often a guise that falls away once the patient is back in the lay world among friends and relatives.

It is in telling the incident to others that the patient's unvoiced thoughts and feelings can be brought to the fore and stressed. The patient can give an account that in her terms is a fuller and more complete picture. The events are embellished with opinions and judgements which at the time of the consultation may have been introspective, or were perhaps not even formulated until after the event when there has been time to make sense of and evaluate what had happened.

In the following excerpt from a woman's report of her consultation with the doctor, we see not only the way in which the teller shows herself dominating the exchange, and the way in which her opinions and feelings about the doctor and the interaction assume prominence, but also something of the process of story-making. The actor in this case leaves the 'acting field', goes over the encounter in her mind and then reconstructs and recounts the incident to her husband when she arrives home. His reaction may also have provided further material for the story which was told to us a few days later.

> . . . he said 'I'm giving you some ointment and some tablets'. I said 'What are the tablets for doctor?' And he said 'To ease the pain', 'Oh well, I don't want tablets for the pain, it's not that bad.' 'Oh all right' he said. You see, if I hadn't asked him, I wouldn't have known if these tablets were for blood pressure or not. I had to ask him if my blood pressure was all right. I'm not bothered about the pain, because it's not that bad. So then the interview was over as far as he was concerned. But I wasn't at all satisfied. I said 'Well what about these dizzy spells I've been having doctor?' And he just sat back and looked at me in silence, staring into my face — thinking of something to say I suppose. So to help him I said 'Do you think it could be my age?' because whatever you've got wrong with you past the age of thirty-five it's always your 'age' and he paused and said 'Well let's put it this way, none of us is getting a day younger are we?' Very profound, I thought. . . . Well, I left the doctor's feeling I just needn't have bothered going. I was thoroughly dissatisfied and I'm none the wiser. . . . When I got home my husband was fuming. He said 'Why do doctors

always treat you as though you've got no intelligence — why should you have to ask what those tablets were, why couldn't he have told you?'

We thus see in the story and the story-telling situation an opportunity for redressing the inequality between the doctor and the patient. Rather than the patient showing herself to others as passive in the face of the doctor, her activity and integrity are stressed, while the conflict and criticisms that were not voiced to the doctor are voiced to relatives and friends.

We have shown how the patient is portrayed in the stories. How is the doctor portrayed? As we might expect, we find that in the critical story the doctor loses the respect that his status might usually afford him. In the story above, for example, we are presented with a rather 'dull' doctor, who is depicted as having to 'think of something to say' and who makes statements which cause the patient to sarcastically muse 'very profound'. Consider, too, the phrases 'pooving around the room' and 'like a nervous rabbit' in the following account. The teller is describing a visit to a gynaecologist to discuss possible infertility.

> I explained to him that I hadn't had a period for some time and could this be anything to do with it and he said he'd do a lot more tests. When I went back for the results a fortnight later I knew what he was going to tell me because there he was, this doctor, pooving around the room sort of hopping from one foot to another like a nervous rabbit. And he finally said: 'Eh — I'm afraid to have to tell you Mrs Brown our tests have shown you're three months pregnant' — I was two months pregnant when they told me I was infertile!

And another person giving a critical account of a doctor:

> I called him in. She had what I thought was chicken pox. And he stood there with his backside in front of the fire, and she was on the settee. 'Well it could be chicken pox' he said.

The image aroused is in direct contrast to that normally associated with a doctor and a professional. A doctor is not normally described as 'like a nervous rabbit' and attention is not normally drawn to his 'backside'. Those who are relatively powerless in a situation can redress the imbalance by stressing their own human and sensible qualities as against the comic qualities or stupidity of the more powerful, in this case the doctor. By laughing at the professional, he is degraded. Similarly, the doctor is often made out to be insensitive or inhuman:

> I was annoyed with our own doctor, we kept the truth from my mother and the callous bugger stood in the passage one day when she called him in and he said, 'Of course you know, you haven't got him much longer, you know what he's got don't you.' 'No,' she said, 'I've got no idea.' 'Well, he's got cancer, and there's nothing you can do for him.'

It is not the particular characteristics of the doctor that determine this portrayal. The same doctor may be portrayed in different ways in different stories. His manner is interpreted to fit the story. The 'charm' of the doctor in one story may be his 'slyness' in another. The 'handsome doctor' in a story of praise may be the 'one who fancies himself with the women' in another. The doctor can also be put down by leaving out the customary title 'Dr' when referring to him.

The inequality between patient and doctor is also redressed when the patient mimics the doctor. Mimicry is used in the tone of the voice of the teller when repeating phrases the doctor was reported to have said. It is used to describe a manner that, for example, is perceived as arrogant, patronising, superior or merely dull. The written transcripts of the tapes we collected fail to bring across this colourful way in which the stories were told. Also mimicked is the way in which certain essential aspects of the doctor's work are carried out. The use of nicknames may draw attention to this. A doctor is meant to give time to his patients: we heard of a doctor who had earned a reputation among his patients for conducting his consultations at great speed and was known as 'two-minute Todd'. A doctor is not meant to take sexual advantage of his patients: in one story a doctor was called 'the Stripper' because of his supposed predilection for internal examinations of his female patients. He can also be mimicked by describing his job as being carried out in an offhand manner. A doctor is meant to take care in examination and diagnosis: one woman described her doctor's 'kerbside manner' saying when he visited at home he would stand at the door rather than examine her children. A doctor is meant to know his treatments: a critical story told to us depicted the doctor asking the patient to pick out from a book the name of the drug he had previously been prescribed.

We would argue that the doctor is necessarily depicted in this way to complement the picture painted by the teller of the patient as sensible, rational, knowledgeable and active. The sharp contrast between the way in which the doctor and the patient are portrayed illustrates how conflict between the lay and medical world is expressed. It is a further way in which the inequalities between doctors and patients can be redressed by the patient.

The reconstruction of encounters between patients and doctors through the medium of the story thus depends as much on the shared opinions and assumptions of the lay teller and the audience about the social world of patients and doctors as it does on the recall of the details of the original exchange. This is why we chose to use the term 'account' to describe the process of describing these events, rather than a term such as 'recall' which capitalises on notions of validity. It was only in looking at the process of consultation, where we gathered material from people at different stages and over time, and used a variety of techniques to gather material, that we were able to compare our own account of the consultation with the accounts given by people in everyday talk.

# 8  The Management of a Therapeutic Encounter

## by Alan Davis and Philip Strong

INTRODUCTION

Different forms of medical treatment require different kinds of co-operation and involvement from the patient. Successful occupational and physiotherapy normally demand the patient's active co-operation with the therapist, whereas, for example, surgery may require only initial assent. This chapter contains a brief analysis of some of the interactional problems encountered by therapists in a children's hospital, and the kinds of solutions they routinely devised. It is based on observational work[1] carried out in three different settings: a physiotherapy department, an occupational therapy department and an orthoptic clinic. The physiotherapists' work comprised treatment of ward in-patients, for such things as chest drainage and limb manipulation, and out-patient treatment of long-term handicapping conditions such as cerebral palsy and spina bifida. The occupational therapists also saw cases of cerebral palsy and spina bifida but concentrated more on arm and hand involvement, as opposed to work on legs and hips. They also treated a few mentally retarded children and psychiatric cases, the latter constituting a third of their referrals. Finally, the orthoptist, who unlike the others also handled adult patients, dealt mainly with the treatment of strabismus (squints). Mentally retarded children were a rarity at the orthoptic clinic.

Work with young or subnormal children is of particular interest in studying how patient involvement is rooted in therapy or other medical treatment. For here the normal rationale that is invoked to justify medical action, and to motivate any necessary client participation — the appeal to 'illness', 'scientific medicine' and the 'normal' desire to 'get better' — is not available to the professional since it is not available to the client. Compliance must, therefore, be sought by other means, and it is these that are explored in this chapter. Since it analyses a situation in which the *normal* assumptions about patients do not apply, it may also serve to clarify those assumptions, for they are often taken for granted. The chapter is also about children and the way adults interact with them, both somewhat neglected topics in sociology.

Our analysis draws mainly on the work of Goffman (1961, 1972a) and of the ethnomethodologists such as Garfinkel (1967) and Cicourel (1973). Both have produced languages in which to talk about interaction, and their work may be very crudely summarised as stating that 'successful' interaction (in the technical sense) requires all parties to be able to define the encounter as of a known sort, and of a beneficial sort. The ethnomethodologists have stressed the constant interpretive task that faces individuals. They have both to work out and to demonstrate that which is going on, namely what is said or thought to be going on. They must continually ground the background rules in concrete behaviour, demonstrating to their own and others' satisfaction that they are oriented to the same features. Thus, in the terms of our chapter, being a doctor, a therapist or a patient is not something that you just passively *are*, it is something that you have to *do*, something that has to be managed or pulled off.

## CHILDHOOD COMPETENCE AND INCOMPETENCE

Everyone in our society is a 'patient' at times and is, therefore, called upon to do patient-work. But as all medical staff know, not everyone can. Young children, those from very different cultures and the insane may lack or fail to exhibit the appropriate cultural competence required of such an identity.

It is an everyday assumption that, because illness is a bad state, people who are 'ill' will wish to get 'better', because to do so is by definition 'better' than being ill. Thus, those who do not appear to want to get better are 'obviously' suffering from abnormal motivation, and lay thought then appeals to 'psychological' disturbances. Parsons (1964) draws on such assumptions in his formulation of the 'sick role'. However, he then uses them to create a harmonious model in which conflict is eliminated. We argue that medical interaction with young children presents special problems. However, we do not mean to imply that, by contrast, interaction with normal adults who are possessed of everyday medical knowledge such as the above is normally a trouble-free enterprise. On this point see for example Horobin and Bloor (1975).

However, very young children or those who are severely handicapped may not know that they are handicapped, may be unaware that potentially better states exist and may, therefore, lack any motivation to get 'better'. They may hate hospitals and define medical staff as people who do pointlessly nasty or incomprehensible things to them. Of course, it could be that some such children are well aware of these things but were routinely treated by medical staff as if they were not and could not be.

Therapists distinguished between two different classes of children. First there were young children of normal intelligence, who were held to be incapable of understanding a medical schema because of their age. Only at around the age of five to six might it first be used, and even then its use was rare and occurred only under provocation.

Second there were retarded children. For those held to be only moderately affected, an appropriate reduction was made to arrive at their 'real' mental age. For the severe cases the problem was, could they understand anything at all? There were no recognised procedures for this; therapists, like parents, fluctuated in their opinion, and there always seemed to be evidence that could be read in either direction. However, such children were routinely classified with the very young.

In either case therapists had to make their activities meaningful to the child and had to create the same involvement in and commitment to the therapy that they might expect the medical schema to create in adults. They coped by appealing to that background knowledge about children that adults in our culture are expected to share. We shall argue that this knowledge contains a central ambiguity about children's 'essential nature', and this ambiguity is reflected in the way they were handled and talked about by therapists.

On one hand the world of children is often portrayed as an essentially different one from that of adults. Play is commonly held to be a constitutive part of a child's identity. Thus, adults in our society 'know' that even if a child cannot do anything else it can always play; and to understand why this is so we must first comprehend what is meant by play. Babies who lack any social competences whatsoever and are thus in a sense non-persons can still be said, quite properly, to play. As the Opies (1967, 1970) have shown, children in our culture have created their own self-sustaining culture of play with its own membership rules and activities. In such a culture children can learn to play social games as equals. It is open to any child to be a competent member and to demand by right that he be treated fairly and according to the rules.

On the other hand adults routinely treat children as not merely incompetent within the terms of their own adult world but as subordinate to them. The world of childhood in this model is not separate and equal but an inferior early stage from which one progresses to adulthood. Children are defined as 'learners', and since adult life is complex they have a lot to learn. They have to learn what sorts of things there are available to be done in the world, the regulative rules for each of these activities, the sorts of people who do them and their reasons for such actions, and the practical ways of recognising, doing and being each of these things (Mead, 1934).

When they are treating children, therapists can, therefore, appeal to either of these models or, as often happens in practice, to both simultaneously. But adults often view play as part of the serious business of learning about life, and one of the tasks of the occupational therapists was to teach mothers not to see their retarded children as 'lazy' and only capable of 'just play', but to view their activities as constructive learning, as an exploration of the world. Seen this way games can be made to serve other purposes besides their own intrinsic rewards. Primary school children may use games to display their various talents, while parents and adults may attempt to intervene in a child's play and guide it in directions which they think most fit. Teaching young children through play is now commonly felt to be the ideal solution to the same educational problems, and in line with this therapists routinely sought to translate their purposes into play — 'It looks like play and it is — but it's play with a purpose.'

For the staff this was a routine solution. New members who often had done most of their training with adults found children's work 'completely different' at first but soon learned to cope, as the practice of this solution to the interpretive problem was a constant topic of conversation and analysis. Therapeutic journals report on the latest transformation attempts, being full of ingenious ideas and elaborate equipment. Professional prestige accrues to those who can most adequately solve the transformation problem. Although we argued earlier that in some sense all children could be held capable of play, in practice therapists were uncertain as to whether severely retarded children could do this. On one occasion a child was described by a therapist as engaging in 'repetitive play' but on another she commented: 'most subnormal children who like playing with water, play with boats or pour water in a funnel. . . . Arthur does not play, he just likes to feel the water.' This seemed to mean that some children were incapable of playing any sustained game with another, or even by themselves. If children could not even play, then therapy was of little or no practical use but was done, if at all, merely to comfort the parents.

Finally, although some therapists said that ideally they would like all their patients to see treatment as play, they seemed in practice not to describe it as such to the children. Therapeutic activities were often presented in game-like forms but the terms 'game' and 'play' themselves were reserved for other occasions, for those times when patients were allowed to play their own games, or when they were held to be not carrying out the therapy properly but merely indulging in 'fun and games'. In fact, apart from the orthoptist no one seemed to have a general term to describe the therapeutic activities to the child. Instead, children were invited to 'throw the ball', 'stand on the board', 'pile these blocks', that is, to take part in activities that could be read as games but were not stated openly to be so. This is not surprising. The medical framework of therapeutic terminology is not used, while if 'play' was extended to cover the therapy, therapists would be unable to discriminate for the children between 'messing about' and the serious matters at hand.

### THERAPEUTIC IDENTITIES

Therapists had difficulty in presenting a therapeutic identity to other medical personnel, to parents, and in particular to the children because of their recourse to 'play' rather than to overt medical treatment in order to accomplish their objectives. Therefore, therapists took considerable trouble to spell out to other medical staff that they were in the business of *treating patients* and not playing with children. They stressed their professional competence in many ways, such as by adopting a highly technical vocabulary with medical superiors and inferiors, while reserving rights to joke about 'playing' for equals and people who 'understood' what therapy is about. These were mainly other therapists.

As well as asserting competence, the therapists also had to acquire the necessary licence to treat the patients. While the medical status of their work was legitimated by the actions of doctors who through referrals created a medical licence to work with the child, the therapist in many ways depended on the co-operation of the parents in creating, sustaining and reinforcing the therapeutic agenda. The therapeutic agenda underlying seemingly trivial activities — such as by getting the child to wear a toy watch on a weak left arm to encourage movement — was explained to parents by showing how the 'work' of the parents complemented that of the therapists, and by dropping their therapeutic identity in favour of a friendly, concerned manner, encouraging parents to feel they could 'really' talk to the therapists in a way that they could not with doctors.

How then did the therapist present herself to the child, and how did she achieve the co-operation of the child? The therapeutic encounter was limited in time and did not have the all-encompassing nature of the family in defining reality for the child. Also, therapy had to begin quickly and was a serious business. The therapist could not rely on direct command alone and had to be judicious in the use of sanctions. She had to find an identity to enable her to involve the child quickly, which required minimal use of sanctions, allowed the child to define the situation as pleasurable, pleased the parents and did not cause trouble with the doctors. It was a game framework that enabled the therapist to solve these problems.

Once established, it allowed other aspects in the relationship to develop over time. Many children eventually showed great affection for their therapist and resented being taken away at the end of the treatment session. Therapists, too, developed attachments to particular children, and these personal ties could be mobilised at a later stage, such as by threatening to withdraw, in order to control the child's misdemeanours. Generally, children seemed to define the treatment situation as pleasurable and perhaps this is not surprising, since in therapy they were the sole focus of the therapists' attention for the one-half to three-quarters of an hour of the treatment. However, despite these attractions, the game framework itself generated a series of interactional problems which the competent therapist had to master in order to bring off a successful treatment session. Before diagnosing the problems, we need to consider the relevant aspects of the medical work in which the therapists engaged.

## THERAPEUTIC AGENDAS

Underlying any treatment session was a 'hidden agenda' (Scheff, 1968) to which the therapist worked and which was often written in the child's record. These agendas required the therapist to move through a repeated set of activities which were designed to bring into action, and in sequence, various muscle groups to enable the child to function as normally as possible. In spina bifida or cerebral palsy, the extent to which normal muscle and limb function can be attained varies. The sequencing of activities was important in that the objective was to take children through developmental stages, adding new ones once the child had achieved some muscle or limb function.

While the underlying rationale, the acquisition of basic motor competences, made sense to the parents and other medical personnel, the mode of its accomplishment with a young child was problematic. The game framework allowed the therapeutic agenda to be hidden under a set of games which therapists played with children. This was particularly important in gaining co-operation, for with young children 'active' movements are required. 'Passive' manipulation of limbs by the therapists are a minimum treatment. However, 'active' movements could not be called out by detailing their therapeutic significance to the child: they had to be brought out by covert means. For example, a very young child who was awaiting heart surgery did not perhaps grasp the therapeutic object in breathing exercises before the operation and refused to co-operate. But blowing 'birdies' made of tissue paper around the bedside called out the necessary breathing activities.

We must now distinguish games therapists play with children, or allow the children to play, and those 'games' that have a hidden therapeutic objective. One advantage of the game framework was that it became possible to move between the two without any overt change in the surface activity. Non-therapeutic games also had their place. They could be used on first contact to create the initial background against which the therapist could identify herself as a playmate, and they filled in the time when the child was awaiting therapy or removal from therapy, or in those cases where there was no serious therapeutic rationale for the child's presence. Once therapeutic 'games' were started the play vocabulary was dropped. Nevertheless, ordinary games had their uses in the actual course of therapy as well, usually either as a reward for good work in 'games' or in situations where the child was flagging in involvement and interest. They were also played when the 'game' framework was in danger of collapse, being inserted into the programme if the therapist feared that discrepant definitions of the situation might become apparent, with a resultant 'scene'. Games also provided the necessary set of rules to be appealed to when 'games' were being played. Games were established as *typical* activities into which hidden therapeutic agendas could be inserted without disruption. They were also played when a sequence of 'games' was difficult to create, the therapist inserting a game into the sequence in order to move through her therapeutic agenda of 'games' in good order.

How did the therapist go about creating 'games'? She had to make them suitable for each child's level of competence and progress. In particular, she had to build upon activities that were already available in the child's vocabulary of games. Mothers were questioned to see if the child was doing anything that might be of therapeutic use. On initial and subsequent contact the therapist watched the child to see what it would and would not do, what it could and could not do. Equipment and toys were given to the child to see what use was made of them.

Having established the child's basic vocabulary of games, the therapist then attempted to enlarge this stock in ways that the child found pleasurable, introducing new items of equipment and getting the child to incorporate them into 'games' with her. If children themselves invented therapeutically valid games then they too might be incorporated. As the sequence developed the therapist modified these games with new regulative rules so that the therapy was better served, but the constitutive rules were left intact; and the child was hopefully still able to see it as a game. Successful therapy demanded that as the child's abilities increased new rules were progressively added to each 'game', so that his or her powers were fully stretched. This tricky task required constant negotiation with the child to build it into the treatment repertoire.

In devising 'games' that called out appropriate responses, the therapists relied partly on recipe knowledge of attractive 'games' that had worked in the past. Thus, blowing paper birds for breathing exercises and inserting a doll in the therapist's tunic top for the child to reach up and kiss were recipes handed on for other cases. Piling bricks as a game could become a 'game' by introducing further sets of rules. For example, piling blocks might first be done with a child's 'good' hand, then with its 'bad' hand in order to build a castle, and then the castle could be kicked over using the 'good' and the 'bad' leg alternately. To start again the child could be encouraged to retrieve the bricks using its 'good' hand, but doing this in a sitting position in which it uses its 'bad' hand to prop itself up.

APPLYING THE GAME IN THERAPY

We now turn to some examples of the game framework in use, and the problems of its implementation. To begin with the child was encouraged to apply a game framework to the therapy through equipment being defined as 'toys' and through the setting being defined as one in which it was legitimate for the child to play. Therapists presented themselves as persons interested in the child to the exclusion of all others around them, as friendly and helpful, as facilitators of pleasant games, as constant sources of praise in success and comfort in distress, and so on. In short, they presented themselves as ideal playmates.

After initial assessment therapists spent some sessions reinforcing this set of definitions, playing games that were like games, since they did not have a strict therapeutic agenda. This came later. During these sessions equipment was explored as a source of 'toys', the therapist talked to the child a lot to establish her interest in him, or allowed the child to define topics of conversation if it was able to do so. At this stage children periodically became aware that their parents were absent or found that they did not like the games or setting, but the therapist was now the only person available to provide comfort, amusement and distraction. Trouble usually ensued when the therapist sought to move on to therapeutic 'games' because the game framework might then be breached in a number of ways. Once the therapist started to manipulate games to conform to her hidden therapeutic agenda, there was always a danger that the reality of the 'game' would break down, to present the child with a new situation which he might not be able to define but might feel threatening. What then were these sources of threat to the 'game'?

The setting itself was a source of problems. For example, while some of the therapeutic props were like toys in shape and design, others were not. Also, the setting was a hospital, in which almost everyone wore a uniform. Other children might be present but were not normally available for games with the child, and he could only play with *his* therapist. Other people were continually walking in and out, and in physiotherapy the child had most of its clothes removed.

As we have argued, one of the major uses of applying a game framework is to motivate the child to engage in the therapeutic activities. Therapists continually monitored the child's motivation to determine whether he was 'really' trying or not. One major factor that might affect this was tiredness, and here again the young child was unable to inform the therapist about this. If the child was not co-operating the reasons for it might be sought in 'tiredness', and the child, therefore, was not worked so hard. If the child did not appear tired then it might lead to sanctioning. Either way, the game framework was liable to break down.

Another difficulty lay in sustaining the exclusiveness of the relationship between therapist and child. Games are usually felt not to be exclusive, and anyone can play. The therapist often had to divert the child's attempts to incorporate other people or objects inappropriate to the therapy.

The rules of the 'games' were a further source of trouble. If in front of game rules both therapist and child are equal, how could the therapist change them without losing credibility as a playmate? If the therapist suddenly appealed to her age and status as a warrant to change the rules, then the child might decide he did not want to play anymore. Indirect tactics were used to prevent conflicts over game rules, like suggesting a new 'game' or incorporating a new object or person to head off a direct confrontation and disruption of the game framework.

Because games for two persons usually involve turn-taking and choosing moves, this also could cause impediments to therapy. Therapists continually tried to construct 'games' in which the child made all the moves and took all the turns. The therapist in her role of playmate had to honour turn-taking some of the time, and if the child demanded she take a turn she had to agree or face a possible row about the rules which might reveal that it was not a game at all. The good therapist was one who was able to develop a set of satisfactory 'games' in which she had minimal involvement as a player and maximum involvement as a facilitator of the child's playing.

Therapeutic activity sometimes produced pain and fright; some tasks could be performed only with great difficulty and uncertainty and there was a corresponding difficulty in getting them defined as fun. When pain and difficulty occurred they were treated in either of two ways. First, they might be treated as incidental to the action and not intimately involved *in* it. Since there was always the chance that the child might withdraw co-operation, the usual strategy was to see how much the child would take before withdrawing and then to divert the child with another 'game' as quickly as possible. The second way was to continue with the treatment while relying throughout on praise and reinforcement to retain involvement. This carried more likelihood of the game breaking down and was used only when the therapist was very sure of the child's relationship with her. Surprise and fear were also problematic and might break the game, and yet involuntary correcting movement of muscles and limbs often can be achieved only if the child is suddenly thrown off balance or startled. This could create problems unless it was defined as a game and therefore safe, but as soon as it was seen as safe by the child it lost its therapeutic value. Consequently, new sources of surprise had to be found by varying the routine or inserting a novel item, or even transferring the child to another therapist.

Games are supposed to be sources of pleasure, and players usually continue playing until they become bored or tired. They may also incorporate new features if both parties consent to a change in the rules. From the therapists' point of view this had disadvantages in that their therapeutic programme required a rapid switching of activities in a set order and no elaboration of the games beyond therapeutic necessity. Children soon developed favourites among the 'games' and wanted to play these all the time and not the others. Since participants have to agree on what game is to be played, the child had rights as a player to choose *his* games. If he chose the wrong ones the therapist had to negotiate the therapy session trying all the while to get the child to play therapeutically improving 'games', while recognising that she had to give way on some demands in order to achieve a balance of satisfactions. To do so she had to obtain the child's acceptance that while some 'games' were not much fun, others were and that you had to honour each other's boring as well as exciting games.

Participants' rewards from the 'games' were also problematic as the two participants had different criteria for allocating rewards. The question then arose whether they were, in fact, playing the same game. For example, if the therapist wanted a child to develop grip and throwing action in a weak left hand she might get the child to throw a ball as far as it could in a certain way and then catch it in return. However, children often mistakenly thought that the game was simply to throw the ball as far as possible, while the therapist would reward only therapeutically correct throwing technique. If such a child hung on to his definition he did not get rewards for success but got sanctions instead. Eventually he might refuse to play any more, forcing the therapist into some accommodation of therapeutic and game-generated rewards.

Sanctions, however, raised problems of authority. If the therapist sanctioned the child she did this by reference either to game-rules or to her position as an adult authority. The former were tried first but in a last resort the therapist withdrew from her identity as playmate and became a serious adult who demanded that the child did as he was told. This was always a last resort as it usually fractured the 'game' framework seriously. Interestingly, in physiotherapy severe sanctioning was usually done by a different therapist. Sometimes the child was threatened with its parents, or the therapist herself might become intractable and refuse to 'play', but insist on the performance of therapy with no escape for the child. After such a confrontation, which the therapist almost invariably won, but at a cost, extra dimensions were added to the 'game' framework. There was now a continual threat that the 'game' framework would be withdrawn entirely, with problematic and unpleasant consequences for the child. Even this appeal might on occasions fail and therapy was then held to be impossible. The two models of childhood which we described earlier contain within them definitions of abnormality.

Thus, just as children who would not play were held to be psychiatrically disturbed, so also were children who persistently refused to recognise a properly licensed adult, such as a therapist, as an 'authority'. One six-year-old girl suffering from mild hemiplegia, who was also a day-patient in the child psychiatric unit, persistently disobeyed therapists and was held to be an impossible patient. Werthman (1968) describes the problems created by such children in American schools.

Since sessions were problematic for young children, the sudden withdrawal of a frame that made some sense of what was going on, and the sudden shift in identities, rendered their situation potentially harmful and unpleasant, especially as they were without their parents' protection. Children were often frightened when this happened, and therefore welcomed the offer to carry on in the 'game' framework within the limits imposed by the therapist. Transfer to another therapist, more active cossetting by the therapist or an appeal to the parents were all employed to warm the child back in again, but whatever the costs, at least the seriousness of the enterprise was firmly established.

## WORKERS' PLAYTIME

Since therapy may last for several years, the therapeutic encounter may stabilise as children learn the routines and develop a more intimate relationship with the therapists. Over this period the normal child's comprehension of the adult world is also growing and the therapist can therefore start to use a medical or work framework in addition to the game one. The constant work of therapists with a child suffering from a mild physical handicap may itself create some of the conditions for the relevance of the medical schema. A limb that is not used may be 'forgotten' by its owner who learns to make do in other, often ingenious, ways. By insisting that it be used 'properly' and often exclusively in the 'games', the therapist may create consciousness of the handicap so that it can be dealt with directly. However the game framework is never entirely superseded but is put to rather different uses. Reasons for the routines can be seen in their immediate beneficial effects and in their place in some long-term programme, and so children can be adjured to work hard to achieve 'success'.

Although a game framework was typically used to provide activities with meaning before the transition to a medical model, there were some important exceptions to this rule, and analysis of these suggests that mental age was not the sole criterion used by therapists for the schema's application. Part of the work of the occupational therapists was to educate their patients in the 'activities of daily living'. Thus, they taught physically handicapped children how to eat with a knife, fork and spoon, how to write properly or how to type with a modified typewriter, and how to dress and tie shoelaces. It is harder to turn such activities into games, but this may not be a drawback, in so far as the child is oriented towards the adult world and wishes to attain some of its competences.

The orthoptist's problems in this respect were far more complex. Almost none of his therapeutic routines could be passed off as 'play', but nor could they be seen as estimable adult skills. The clinic was full of technical equipment, and the tasks demanded a very high level of both intellectual competence and motivation to perform a series of complex acts of recognition over a period of fifteen to twenty minutes. This seems to have radically affected the definitional work of the therapist, although since we observed the work of only one orthoptist, this could simply be his particular style. But whatever the causes there were two important differences between the orthoptic and other departments. Unlike the other therapeutic departments we observed, children were exhorted to 'work' from an early age. Unlike other departments, young children were frequently told as soon as they entered the room that of course they could do it because 'You're a big boy now, aren't you'. It seemed that the appeal to a game framework depended not simply on the patient's age but also on the complexity and nature of the task to be performed, and some therapeutic tasks seemed incapable of being successfully transformed into games.

Just as some tasks could not be turned into games, so it was held that some children could not be games-players, so that for them also the game framework was irrelevant. As we have already noted, therapists held that some children were hardly capable of 'play' let alone 'work'. All the therapeutic games demanded active participation from the children and thus a minimum ability to understand and carry out commands. For those who lacked this, therapy in the orthoptic and occupational therapy departments was held to be impossible. The physiotherapists could, however, treat some of these children if they were physically handicapped as well, since part of their work involved 'passive' therapy. Here the child's body was treated as an object to be manipulated by the therapist rather than by the patient. Since such tasks did not require the child's active co-operation there was no need for a games schema to make sense of the activity, and the therapist could use an overtly *clinical* framework.

The game framework therefore could not be applied under all conditions, and even when it seemed appropriate, its use demanded considerable skills from the therapist. We conclude by noting that therapeutic games are not confined solely to young children. With adults there is less of a problem of comprehension of the therapeutic rationale. However, there is a new problem in that they may define such activities as childish and demeaning. Comprehension does not guarantee motivation. Adult paraplegics from all over the world compete in the Paraplegic Olympics in contests such as archery, basketball and swimming, and such games may form a regular part of adult therapy. Similarly, some of the older children we observed found a valuable incentive to effort in therapy in the games and leisure pursuits of the adult world. Some older boys treated the exercises in physiotherapy like gymnastics as occasions for demonstrating their bodily skills and strength. A ten-year-old girl in occupational therapy who had consistently failed to wear a corrective splint or carry out her prescribed home exercises suddenly became most keen when a therapist gave her a specially modified sewing-ring and taught her to use it. Such games or pastimes, however, although perhaps therapeutic, are rather different from those that are played with young children, for the patients are *aware* of their therapeutic value. They do not, therefore, act as a framework to make the therapy meaningful, though of course the forms they take may render it more palatable.

NOTE

1 This observational work is part of a larger study carried out by the authors and Heather Gibson into the involvement and treatment of young handicapped children, and financed by the Social Science Research Council as part of a programme grant.

# 9  Please See and Advise: Handling Referrals to a Psychiatric Hospital
## *by David Robinson*

The increase in the numbers of emergency and out-patient clinic attendances in England, America and elsewhere is not new. Nor is the realisation that, in spite of this increase, health surveys still report that large proportions of apparently healthy general population samples have some aberration or disorder considered by medical professionals to be well worthy of attention. These two features of everyday medical life cause much concern among those practitioners and administrators responsible for, or wishing to shape the future of, the medical services. They also raise other issues that require elaboration and elucidation. Two general questions that immediately suggest themselves are first. 'With what criteria do referral agents operate to come to the conclusion that some case is worthy of referral to some specialist medical facility?' and second, 'With what criteria do specialist medical staff operate to decide upon the legitimacy or acceptability of any particular referral?'

The main body of this chapter focuses on the second of these two questions, and discusses referrals to an alcoholism out-patient clinic. Just as 'noticing alcoholism' and 'referring someone to an alcoholism clinic' is not understandable unless placed in the context of ideas about what counts as alcoholism, the range and nature of available help and treatment and the appropriate referral of particular people to particular organisations, so the staff of organisations to which people with drink-related problems are referred have their own ideas about what counts as an appropriate referral, and have routines for handling those referrals that are considered to fall outside this category and for discouraging further referrals of that type.

That alcoholism is messily defined is readily acknowledged by those who work with, study, treat, help, judge or live with people who are considered to have some alcohol-related problem. It is not the sociologist's task, however, to define 'alcoholism' or 'an alcoholic' so that such definitions can be universally applied to indicate diseases to be cured, studied or consulted about, or people to be treated or helped, prosecuted, sympathised with or admired. What a sociologist *can* be expected to do is to describe, attempt to explain and indicate the implications of the fact that people differ systematically in their assessment of what counts as alcoholism, being an alcoholic, normal drinking, drinking problem, treatment, help and so on. For despite the lack of universally accepted definitions, both professionals and laymen do employ the notions 'alcoholism' and 'alcoholic' in the course of their everyday lives. Thus, the parent study (Robinson, 1976) from which the material in this chapter is taken does not focus directly upon the question 'What is alcoholism?', but rather on the question as it is transposed into problems such as 'What is alcoholism taken to mean by particular people in particular situations?' and 'How do some people get into the position in which they are defined, by themselves or by others, as alcoholics?'

REFERRALS AND THE USE OF CASE RECORDS

As part of the study particular attention was focused on the question of referral to the out-patient department of a psychiatric hospital. The aim was to place the discussion of 'What is alcoholism?' within a specific setting in order to see how 'the question of definition' was handled both by those in that setting and by those who made referrals to it. Referral behaviour is of particular research interest since the referral agent does have to, in a sense, come clean about his notions of alcoholism, alcohol-related problems, help or treatment. For 'alcoholism' and 'becoming an alcoholic' are *in essence* that set of practices enforced when people employ such notions in the course of their everyday lives. This is not to say that alcoholism and the alcoholic are not as well a product of biochemical apparatus and processes: they are, of course. But biochemical and physiological states and processes are 'noticed', 'recognise', 'assessed', responded to', 'treated' and so on, and such activities occur in specific social contexts. It is this that gives 'alcoholism' and 'becoming an alcoholic' their distinctly social features.

The following discussion of handling referrals is based almost entirely upon material from the *case notes and records* of people referred with some drink-related problem to Hospital H during one calendar year. In the context of the parent study, the case notes revealed the universe and distribution of referral agencies that advanced patients to Hospital H during that particular period. For, of course, one way of categorising the clientele of an organisation is to consider from where they come. This may seem an obvious thing to do, but it is not insignificant. For as Freidson (1971) reminds us, 'In more cases than may be at first apparent, whether or not one will be diagnosed or treated in a certain way depends in part on what is "actually" wrong and in part on the professional agent one chooses and the referral system in which one is located.' Of the 2,686 new patients registered in the study period, the case records of 207 of them mentioned some drink-related problem. Of those 207, 40 per cent were referred by general practitioners, 20 per cent were self-referrals, while four other small categories — other hospitals, probation service, social work agencies and Alcoholics Anonymous (AA) — accounted for approximately 10 per cent of referrals each.

The fact that as many as one in five of the cases were self-referred is not surprising since the emergency clinic at Hospital H is open twenty-four hours a day; no appointment is needed; if one's case is considered urgent it will be attended to immediately; diagnosis and treatment facilities are at hand; and quick in-patient admission is possible. Indeed, given all this, it is easy to see Roth's (1971) point when he suggests that: '. . . perhaps we should stop asking why people come to an emergency department, and instead ask why anyone gets his care anywhere else'.

But in addition, of course, the accounts of the case, and in particular the correspondence between the referral agents and the hospital staff, were of interest in themselves in that they gave some indication of what information was made available, to whom, and when. For accounts are made and called for when there is thought to be something to be explained. The presence or absence of an expected or requested account indicates the nature of the relationship between the individuals or organisations concerned, since accounts are only given to those to whom we feel accountable.

## HANDLING REFERRALS FROM VARIOUS SOURCES

Referral behaviour is a research topic of interest not only for what it reveals about the referral agent's definition of the problem that is being presented; the act of referral also, by definition, links people together. Thus, 'the act of referral' is also of interest in that it is likely to reveal something of the nature of the relationship between those different sets or categories of people.

From the material in the case notes two simple preliminary facts about handling emerged. First, only five per cent or so of the cases were explicitly rejected. That is, nearly all the cases were accepted, where *accepted* means that Hospital H accepted responsibility for them. Either an in-patient or out-patient treatment programme was initiated or the patient was discharged as not being in need of medical treatment — but that decision was made at Hospital H. The second fact to emerge was that in approximately fifty per cent of the cases that were accepted, the referral agent was discouraged from making further referrals. This was done either by making no reply to the referral letter or by replying and explicitly discouraging further referrals of that type.

In addition, it was clear that whether or not cases were accepted, and whether or not further referrals were discouraged, could *not* be explained in terms of either the agreed *seriousness* of the case or the particular *source* of the referral. Thus, two quite straightforward questions about these referrals are raised.

(i)   Why were certain cases rejected and how were these rejections handled?

(ii)   Why were certain referral agents, both medical and non-medical, discouraged from making further referrals — where *discouraged* means either explicitly discouraged by being rebuked, or implicitly discouraged by not being replied to or corresponded with?

It was suggested earlier that, given estimates of need based upon health survey research, specialist medical facilities are scarce. In the alcoholism services, given current official estimations of the number of alcoholics or people with alcohol-related problems, and the current increase in the likelihood that such people will be considered to have a 'medical' problem, the scarcity of specialist medical facilities is particularly acute. In 1974 there were under four hundred 'alcoholism treatment unit' beds in England for a problem said to affect anywhere between 300,000 and 600,000 individuals. Thus, however the definitional questions in relation to diagnosis are handled, that is 'scarcity of facilities' par excellence. In this situation specialist practitioners are called upon to make routine decisions about which among many suitable cases for in-patient treatment shall receive it. Similarly, since many people recognise and seek advice about their own or other people's alcohol-related problems, decisions have to be made about appropriate channels of referral *to* specialist medical facilities. In short, specialist medical practitioners act as gate-keepers to facilities, in that they must control not only access but the amount and type of contact. This is the nature of the case in *any* specialist medical facility, but appears to be particularly acute in relation to alcoholism.

It could be argued that a major reason why cases in any medical setting are accepted is that the medical professional is *obliged* to accept them, on the grounds that quite simply it is the task of a practitioner to give help when it is needed: it is not a question of choice but one of duty. As the International Code of Medical Ethics puts it, 'A doctor must give care as a humanitarian duty unless he is assured that others are willing and able to give such care.' Clearly, the question of being assured of others' willingness and ability is complex, but the implication is that a medical professional will provide care if it is needed unless it can be guaranteed elsewhere. In the case of people referred for specialist medical attention from non-medical sources this is clearly a consideration of no little

*Handling referrals to a psychiatric hospital*

| Modes of response to referrals | The specialist's obligation | Main sources of referrals | % of all cases (approx.) |
|---|---|---|---|
| A: Accept the referral + Maintain contact with the agent | Controllable obligation | GPs Probation officers (I) | 60 |
| B: Accept the referral + Discourage further referrals from that source | Uncontrollable obligation | Probation officers (II) Alcoholics Anonymous Social workers Other hospitals (I) | 35 |
| C: Reject the referral + Discourage further referrals from that source | No obligation | Other hospitals (II) | 5 |

importance. A second *core* feature of the obligation to accept a case applies specifically to a practitioner in specialist medical settings and is the reciprocal part of one of the basic principles of the Hippocratic Oath, namely that any medical practitioner should 'defer to specialist assistance whenever this is in the best interests of the patient'. Clearly, this has meaning only if specialist practitioners accept the complementary obligation to *provide* that assistance.

In addition to the *obligations* of the medical practitioner in Hospital H, there is an administrative rule in respect of catchment area referrals. Hospital H has an obligation to care for those persons who live within a particular area around the hospital. But this does not mean that referrals cannot be accepted from *outside*. In fact, only about fifteen per cent of referrals to the alcoholism clinic at Hospital H during the study period came from *within* the catchment area.

Given that specialist practitioners have to exercise control over scarce resources, given the nature of medical professional obligations, and given an administrative rule, it was possible to distinguish three typical modes of response, by Hospital H, to referrals from a whole range of medical and non-medical sources. These are set out in the table.

## A: Accept the referral and maintain contact with the agent

The first mode of response was that in which Hospital H accepted the case and maintained some kind of contact with the referral agent. Further referrals were not encouraged — in a situation of scarce resources who would do that? — but further referrals were not *dis*couraged. Most of the cases in this category came from general practitioners. In fact, they represented an easily recognisable common mode of referral; namely of 'a generalist deferring to specialist assistance'. Such assistance may be to confirm 'offered' diagnoses, to provide specialist treatment or to give advice on how the generalist might himself manage the case.

However, the *style* of the referrals and the subsequent correspondence reveal that the specialist practitioner was given a great deal of room for manoeuvre. While the GPs' referral letters might contain a great deal of information and opinion about the cause and consequences of the alcohol-related problems, and often contained detailed statements about the patient's 'motivation for treatment' and explanations of why the referral was made 'at that time', there was rarely any indication of the *type* of treatment that was being sought. The case was in greater or lesser detail described, and then merely presented with a request to 'please see and advise'. Only one letter actually mentioned, and then in only the most broad terms, the *kind* of help that the GP felt was necessary: 'She obviously requires a great deal of help at this stage, and I am sure she should be under observation as an in-patient.'

The hospital staff's room for manoeuvre, therefore, is extensive. In addition, they know that the case can be returned to the care of the GP, who will take up again complete medical responsibility for it. Thus, core obligations are easy to satisfy and only such strain on resources will be exerted as the specialist practitioner sees fit. In such cases the specialist will maintain contact with the referral agent, he will thank him for the referral and in all probability send a letter giving details of diagnosis and treatment, opinion and advice as to future management of the case.

Another set of referrals that came into category A were those cases sent by probation officers in relation to remand requirements at Magistrates' Courts. The correspondence between the probation officer and the specialist in the relatively small number of such cases was open, full and courteous. Both had a part to play *vis-à-vis* the legal process. From the specialist's point of view the procedure — providing a court report — would be circumscribed and short-term, and thus make no great demands upon resources, while the probation officer, unlike the GP, was as likely to offer help as to request it. Again, as with the GP referrals, the specialist practitioner is accepting *controllable* cases, which do not put any strain on resources. However, not all probation office referrals were of this type. Others came into category B, where the nature of the relationship between the officer and the hospital psychiatrist, as revealed by the correspondence, was quite different.

*B: Accept the referral and discourage further referrals from that source*

The nature of the relationship between probation officers and specialists was quite different when patients were referred direct to Hospital H for 'purely medical', as opposed to 'medical-in-a-legal-framework', reasons. In every case the patient was seen and courses of treatment were initiated. The cases were, in a sense, 'unrefusable', in that it was clear that at least certain aspects required medical attention that could *not* be provided by the referring agency. Hospital H was, thus, obliged to accept the case.

Since the cases could not, by definition, be sent back to a referral agent who could accept medical responsibility for them, the specialist practitioner was not so easily able to control the referral situation. The medical buck had stopped there. Clearly, the hospital's ability to control scarce resources would be seriously undermined if this category of cases expanded. Further referrals of this kind were, therefore, discouraged. No replies were sent to the majority of probation officers who referred in this way. In one case a reply *was* sent but only in order to rebuke the referring officer who had sent a patient, with a very short accompanying letter, to the emergency clinic. The referral letter said:

> Mr X has suffered from nervousness for some years now, and finds that the only way he can face a new day and new people is by taking two or three pints of beer. Perhaps you can help him in this matter.

The Duty Registrar replied:

> Thank you for referring this patient who I saw in the emergency clinic on Xth of June. I understand from the patient that his GP did not know that he had been referred here. However, I have sent a full report to him and suggested a course of treatment. I think in future it might be better if you get a patient's GP to refer him/her to Hospital H who can then give us any medical history that we require when seeing the patient.

The point about the 'medical history' is an important one, but the fact remains that the case was immediately taken out of the probation officer's sphere of influence. What his professional relationship with the patient was is uncertain since he didn't reveal it in the short referral letter. However, the reply to the probation officer from Hospital H did not mention the diagnosis, or the course of treatment that had been initiated or other action that had been taken. The isolation of the probation officer from his client was further strengthened when, in the hospital's letter to the patient's GP, the officer was not mentioned by name:

> Dear Doctor X, your patient was referred to us by *a probation*

*officer* at XYZ Magistrates Court and appeared with a letter written two weeks ago. . . .

Interviews with all the probation officers in the study area confirmed how resentful many of them are about information being withheld from them. Comments ranged from the mild —

> . . . psychiatrists could be a little more forthcoming about what they're doing with clients.

via:

> I feel very strongly about not getting information back from other agencies — particularly psychiatrists.

to the officer who complained bitterly of the

> . . . out of date ethics — like psychiatrists only accepting referrals via GPs — it's a waste of time and nonsense, the medical myth and etiquette. Psychiatrists sometimes send back a bald statement about a client, with no explanation, as if they're handing down judgement.

It is hardly surprising that one should say that probation officers 'feel that they are looked down on', or that another should conclude that:

> We should all get our heads together for the good of the individual. But . . . psychiatrists make us work very hard for our referrals, and give very little back. I don't think it's worth the bother.

Other referrals that fell into the 'unrefusable' category were those from AA and from social workers; these were handled in the same way as those from probation officers. Most of the referrals from 'other hospitals' were rejected, and these rejections will be discussed later. However, some referrals from 'other hospitals' *were* accepted.

It could be argued that one hospital with scarce facilities can pass a patient to another hospital with scarce facilities only if it is able to make the case either very attractive or unrefusable. It will be seen later how attempts to make cases attractive failed. However, some referrals were 'successful', and these were the ones in which the referring hospital demonstrated a clear lack of ability to deal with the case itself. One resulted from a 'very difficult' situation in which 'Neither Mrs X nor her husband speak English, although her daughter gave me a reasonable history. Mrs X is now a little paranoid in her attitude so that she wishes to be seen alone, which means that her only daughter is precluded from interpreting for her, consequently everyone is anxious that she should be seen by a German-speaking psychiatrist in the hope that this may prove helpful.' In short, the case was unrefusable in that Hospital H was obliged to accept it on the grounds that it could not be assured that others, while they may have been *willing*, were *able* to give the care that was needed.

The other referrals from 'another hospital' that succeeded did so because they were made 'across-specialties'. For example, a consultant chest physician working in a chest clinic wrote in detail about his successful treatment of a patient's tuberculosis. The TB treatment began in 1959, and in recent years

> . . . he has kept fairly well as far as his chest is concerned and his tuberculosis has shown no signs of reactivating; his last X-ray here was on 23rd April. . . .

The letter then went on to describe the fact that the patient

> . . . has always been a heavy drinker and has smelt of alcohol on many occasions when he attended the clinic. He admitted in 1965 to drinking 14 pints of beer a day . . . . [the referral to the alcoholism clinic was made several years later] . . . he has been unemployable for many years and has let himself deteriorate very badly. He now admits to spending every penny that he can on drink. . . . I would appreciate anything you can do for him.

Again, this could be described as an unrefusable case in that it could not be assumed that it could be handled where it was. Further contact was discouraged in that no reply was sent to the referral agent. All other referrals from 'other hospitals' were rejected and come into the next category.

## C: Reject the referral and discourage further referrals from that source

The third category is made up of those small number of referrals that were explicitly rejected. All of them came from 'other hospitals'. It could be argued that if specialists are gate-keepers to scarce medical facilities then they are most likely to reject cases that they are not obliged — as defined previously — to accept. The rejected referrals from 'other hospitals' were without exception more serious in terms of reported problems and prognosis than those that were accepted. In one case, for example, the referring hospital described in detail the social, physical, and psychological deterioration of the patient and concluded that:

> He is a pleasant enough chap who freely admits and discusses his problem and I think sincerely wants a cure. From his recent record I think this will only be possible with prolonged specialist treatment which we are not really able to give. . . .

The letter adds, as a final piece of evidence as to the seriousness of the case, that:

> If he does not stop drinking now, his prognosis from the point of view of his liver is obviously very poor, and one might expect him to live another five years.

The reply from Hospital H, after the single out-patient visit, repeated the details about the seriousness of the condition and concluded that:

> . . . as you suggest, it seems imperative now that he should undergo a period of in-patient investigation and management, preferably in a specialised setting.

but added that:

> Unfortunately, our waiting list here is fairly long, and since he does not live within the hospital catchment area, I cannot see a bed becoming available within the next two months.

and suggested to the referring hospital that:

> . . . if you could, therefore, explore the local services, then this might be the best policy.

As a concession the letter ended by saying that Hospital H had:

> . . . put his name on the waiting list, and it can certainly stay there if there are no alternatives available.

Thus, the referral failed. It might be said that the case was over-sold, in that, by pressing it as extremely urgent, it meant that, in fact, immediate admission was being asked for. The impression was certainly given that immediate admission was considered to be the only possible course of action. However, once the 'waiting list' response was made by Hospital H, backed up by the catchment area rule, the referring hospital's ploy had failed. Even the waiting list 'offer' could hardly be accepted, since that would have been tantamount to admitting that the case was not as urgent as had been suggested. As in all bargains and exchanges the higher the stakes the greater the setback if a move fails.

In a situation in which it is legitimate to pass the case back — because there is specialist cover at the referring hospital — it is difficult to see how a successful referral could be made, especially in cases when the catchment area rule can be invoked as well. This is not to say, of course, that if we know where the patient lives we should be able to predict whether or not a referral will be accepted. Since only fifteen per cent of patients seen at the alcoholism clinic at Hospital H came from within the catchment area this is obviously not so. But in any case, rules do not work in that way. They do not control action. They are not disembodied standards, but human arrangements to be invoked and pressed in particular situations. As Strauss (1964) succinctly puts it:

> Rules enter into current and future conduct in that actors define rules as relevant to situations, which means that they must define situations as related or unrelated to specific governing rules. Consequently . . . people expect rules to control their own and others' behaviour. They also counter others' claims to be rule-appliers with claims of their own.

CONCLUSION

This chapter has presented material from a study of drinking and alcoholism, and particular attention has been focused on the case notes of people referred to a psychiatric out-patient department. The act of referral plays an important part in the process of being diagnosed as, or coming to take oneself to be, an alcoholic. In addition, referral behaviour is of particular research interest since the referral agent does have to, in a sense, come clean about his idea of what counts as alcoholism, an alcohol-related problem, an appropriate referral and the appropriate time for making it.

But any attempt to explain why referral agents do what they do must also be informed by a consideration of the activities and practices of those to whom they have referred in the past, or might be likely to refer in the future. Referral agents will be to a greater or lesser extent aware of the ideas that the staff who control scarce resources have about 'what counts as' an appropriate referral. Similarly, they will have either experienced or not experienced those procedures for handling referrals that are considered to be inappropriate. For if we are to understand social action in any situation we must attempt to tease out the rules that are taken by particular categories of people as justifications for action, and to explain why certain people's claims to be rule-appliers are more successful than other people's.

David Goldberg (1972), writing about psychiatry in general practice, claims that 'GPs only refer one in twenty of their disturbed patients to a psychiatrist', and suggests that 'if they were only slightly less selective in their referrals, the out-patient service would be brought to its knees'. It could be argued that just as important in any explanation of why out-patient services are not 'brought to their knees' is the specialist medical practitioner's ability to discourage 'uncontrollable' or 'unrefusable' referrals.

# Professional Ideology
# and Mental Illness

# 10 The Production and Management of Stupidity: The Involvement of Medicine and Psychology

## by Joanna Ryan

This chapter presents a mixture of conceptual, historical and political observations about the way our society (mostly England and America) deals with stupidity and in particular about the role of psychology in this. I write as a critical psychologist, trying to make sense of the concepts and categories presented in psychological and medical books on the subject and of their relation to the practices and institutions around us. Psychology is involved in stupidity in a multitude of ways: in the 'caring' and 'knowledge' industries, in medicine, and in education, as an apparent bridge between the biological and the social. It has played a crucial instrumental role in providing the technology for various practices, but it has also had a relatively low status, especially in the eyes of doctors and psychologists in other fields.

Stupidity[1] is about the lowest status of all disabling and disqualifying conditions (e.g. Wilson, 1970). The ultimate, if not most important, stigma is its exclusion from Goffman's (1963) book, *Stigma*, except for a footnote. Most of the readers of this chapter, if they have not had occasion to think about the subject, will probably feel a mixture of indifference, disgust and guilt about it. Stupid people, if they are not so low-grade as to horrify, are usually boring, especially to intellectuals. It is not so easy to glorify stupidity as it is madness, or to see the definitions as only those of social deviance and non-conformity. Although there is scope for much greater cultural relativism than is usually appreciated, especially in relation to how the stupid are treated (Edgerton, 1970, provides the only useful review on this subject), this does not mean

153

there will be no stupid people in an ideal society or that differences in competence will cease to be socially meaningful. Every society for which there is information has its inept people. Societies vary, however, in their ideas of what skills are regarded as socially desirable, how these skills are acquired and what social support there is for those who, for whatever reason, cannnot acquire them.

Trying to understand how our society has got into the mess it has — as regards the numbers defined as subnormal, the stigma and the actual conditions of existence of so many of them — can clarify our thoughts about what ought to happen in the future. I have found most psychological work on the subject extremely confusing in this respect since it evades, while appearing to grapple with, most of the fundamental questions. It performs this mystification within the historical context of medical hegemony of the whole field of stupidity. This chapter tries to examine the reasons for its location there. The currently increasing 'educational' influences, often seen as oppositional to medical ones, will also be considered.


MEDICAL CONTROL

A brief outline of the history of medical involvement in subnormality will provide a context for later discussion of the domination of psychology by medical concepts. Pritchard (1963) and Kanner (1964) provide more detailed chronological accounts of the main developments. The origins of Western philanthropic concern with idiots are usually located in France towards the end of the eighteenth century. Most of the early pioneers were doctors (Pereire, Itard, Seguin) who often had experience of institutions for the blind and deaf-mute. However, their aims and their subsequent influence are commonly regarded as 'educational', in that they emphasised 'scientific' methods of training and improvement and the eventual return to independent living. The first institute for the education of cretins, set up in Switzerland in 1841, was also founded by a doctor (Guggenbuhl). This too had ambitious educational aims. The 1840s saw the founding of the first English institutions, influenced initially by continental ideas. These had doctors at their head, as did the much larger asylums for the mentally deficient that proliferated in the second half of the nineteenth century. It was not until the turn of the century that special classes and schools were created within the educational system, and here again doctors and other medical personnel seem to have been instrumental in pressing for their establishment. The subcommittee of the Charity Organisation Society, which strongly advocated the creation of special classes, had only medical and no educational representatives. The procedures for selection for special schools, and for exclusion from education altogether, gave doctors most — usually sole — power in the decisions. The 1944 Education Act still gave medical personnel some say in selection for special schools, and a doctor's signature was required for exclusion from education. Until 1970 local health authorities ran the training centres for those excluded from education. Now, no child is considered administratively ineducable, so that all children of school age, whether in hospital or not, are theoretically the responsibility of a local education authority.

The large public asylums that were established in the late nineteenth century were from the beginning under medical direction. Some formal education was provided for some of the children, as was occupational training for the more promising adults. But, although the early institutions had been set up in an era of educational optimism, with the explicit aim of returning people to society, they increasingly became regarded as life-time custodial institutions. The eugenic scare of the early twentieth century, and the alarms about the supposed social inadequacy and danger of the deficient, confirmed and reinforced this pre-existing trend. The invention of intelligence tests (*c.* 1908), with the idea of fixed individual potential, led to the 'discovery' of many more defectives than had been thought to exist. The function of asylums was increasingly seen as protecting society rather than catering for the needs of individual inmates. In terms of buildings and traditions, this is the legacy we are now left with, although the ideology has changed.

Why did the medical profession have such extensive control over the provision of care and training for the subnormal? This is an important question, since it has been repeatedly shown that the majority of subnormal patients actually in hospitals do not require any medical or nursing care, and that many more require only simple assistance (e.g. Leck *et al.*, 1967; King *et al.*, 1971). The proportion of those not requiring medical care must have been even greater in the past, when the most chronically and multiply handicapped were less likely to survive than they are now. Sociological studies (e.g. King *et al.*, 1971) have shown how unsuited hospital regimes even in the 'best' hospitals are to child care, and how the training of nurses and doctors is quite inappropriate to the care of those who are not ill. Since it is clear that what medical care has provided for the stupid is not in their best interests or particularly suited to their needs — indeed, is now an unmitigated disaster — it is extremely important to answer the question posed at the head of this paragraph. Perhaps answers will be found in a general consideration of how medicine is used to deal with social misfits of all kinds, and of how medical institutions have been and are used as prisons and dumping grounds for various kinds of undesirables.

A detailed historical and political study of the rise of subnormality institutions of the kind that has been partially provided for madness is needed to answer these questions. Speculative thoughts are offered on the background to the rise of medical institutions for the subnormal, especially the changes in social and family relations caused by the development of industrial capitalism throughout the nineteenth century.

Radical changes in labour requirements demanded, among other things, a labour force with skills that could not be learned in the family or neighbourhood. Factory processes had to be learned in the factory, and reading and writing at school — universal compulsory education was established in 1870. There were also many attempts to impose greater discipline and speed on the work force, while increasing stratification of the work force meant greater divisions and specialisations of skills, especially managerial and clerical ones.

It is often argued that it is the technological complexity of modern society that has created the enormous social problem of mental subnormality — a problem that can only increase as society 'advances' and the minimum requirements for independent living become beyond the reach of more and more people. A contrast is usually drawn with unspecified primitive or simpler societies where, it is alleged, the demands of life are such that many people (the mildly subnormal of our society) are not even recognised as incompetent, and the severely subnormal either do not survive or are tolerated and given some kind of socially acknowledged function. This 'simple people for simple societies' view, apart from displaying the worst ethnocentrism characteristic of much of American sociology, is both unfounded empirically and also seriously misleading in seeing technological change as the only or crucial determinant of how many people are regarded as subnormal.

All societies for which there is evidence recognise some of their members as incompetent, but they differ greatly as to how they treat such people and in the extent to which they are a problem. Edgerton (1970) argues that no cross-cultural generalisation is possible about the relationship of this to economic factors or the mode of survival in a particular society since the variety is so great. He also points out that many of the skills needed in 'simple' societies are in fact very complex in the demands they make on an individual's flexibility and independence, and that they may take years of initiation and learning to acquire. The argument about technological change is misleading because it ignores the fact that many advanced technological processes, for example repetitive 'unskilled' factory work, are in fact extremely simple to carry out and are often simpler than those traditional or craft skills that they replace. Other social changes that accompany major technological changes are probably more crucial in determining how incompetent or other marginal people can survive in a society.

Throughout the nineteenth century, as more and more people were drawn into factories, extremely far-reaching changes took place affecting the relationship between home and work, the stability of family life, the status of women, the increasing state control of education and its removal from the family. When production was mostly domestic, with all the family involved, the necessary skills would have been acquired in the family. As production was increasingly removed from the family, and the family systems of apprenticeship and work allocation in factories disappeared, the educative role of the family was increasingly taken over by other agencies. It does not seem unreasonable to suppose that opportunities to learn useful skills were thereby diminished for those who were already slow to learn. Families are likely to have been more flexible in the provision of possible roles for the stupid and to have taken more time in teaching them skills, than a factory with its concern with efficiency and profitability. It would also have been more in the family interests to have taken trouble in this way, since they did not have the cheap and expendable pool of labour available to replace deficient members that the factory owners had, and still do have.

This factor of time and speed is extremely important in many other ways. One of the major needs of developing capitalism was for a well disciplined work force, and one of the respects in which greater discipline was (and still is) required was increased speed on production lines. This concern with speed is reflected in many aspects of our education system, and it works to the disadvantage of the stupid. When elementary education was first instituted there was great concern for drawing up standards for educational progress within a school. Indeed, classes were first of all named 'standards', and it was eventually stipulated that no child should remain in one standard for more than a certain number of years, the norm being one. Thus, school achievement and educational progress were defined and measured in terms of the rate of acquisition of certain skills. The invention of intelligence tests and the idea of IQ was the next logical step, in that the stupid were actually and officially defined in terms of a rate measure — rate of change of mental age with chronological age. The stupid are those who do not change quickly enough along a particular dimension. The most intelligent are those whose rate of change of mental age with chronological age is fastest. (See Ryan, 1972, for a fuller explication of the construction of this rate measure.) Psychologists in their endless wonderings about what intelligence really is, or what IQ really means, have concentrated entirely on the supposed cognitive aspects, such as the ability to reason, learn and judge. They have completely ignored the essential quantitative speed of development aspect. But this speed aspect is vitally important, for it is actually in terms of the amount of time they have to spend attaining the same level of competence as much younger children that the stupid are defined.

The ultimate irony is that it took psychology until the 1950s to discover that even the severely subnormal were in fact capable of being trained to perform various kinds of industrial tasks — the crucial factor being in most cases not any inability to learn the task, but simply the time and methods taken to do so. Sufficiently detailed specification of all aspects of the task in question, and adequate practice at all stages of learning, produced levels of final performance that were satisfactory for the task in question. Subsequent work on learning, visual discrimination, memory and reaction times have underlined this conclusion, that a person's apparent inability to learn is, to a much greater extent than usually acknowledged, a function of the time allowed for him to learn. Such findings are only 'discoveries' in a context that denies their possibility. Thus it is not changes in the technological sophistication of production processes that lead to the creation of increasing numbers of subnormals, but the various changes in social relations that these technological changes are part of, and that make it more difficult for the relatively stupid to acquire any socially useful skills. The educational agencies that are allegedly designed to help them to do so tend to exacerbate the problem by adopting many of the same criteria of efficiency that capitalist production does.

The cost of so many marginal people is borne by the family and the State. The benefits accrue mostly to employers, and to those who are employed and make a profession of looking after the subnormal. It is well known that the success rate of hospitals in releasing their patients, and the patients' viability in the community, depends largely on the prevailing level of unemployment (Farber, 1968). Despite such findings, the idea that the subnormal are a surplus population, available in times of labour shortage but expendable otherwise, has not gained much attention from psychologists. Instead they seem more attracted by the idea currently purveyed by Jensen (1970) and others, that the subnormal are *necessarily* an unproductive group and an economic burden on society, because of their limited learning ability. Such a position prefers to see psychological descriptions and definitions of people's abilities as absolute and inevitable and as the only relevant descriptions.

It is also important to consider what system of social support there is, or could be, in any society for those who are in some way dependent — children, old people, the incompetent. In our society the isolation of the nuclear family puts immense strains on any family that has dependants, even where these are young 'normal' children, let alone the old, the sick or the crazy. There are many studies demonstrating the extraordinary domestic strains, especially on the mother, of subnormal dependants (see, for example, Bayley, 1973). It is very important to speculate on how family and community life could be different in these respects, because apparently small changes could have far-reaching implications for the viability of the incompetent and a sharing of the 'problem', and such changes would not present an impossible burden for any one person or make life intolerable for the dependent person in question. For example, suppose public transport really was public transport. If conductors on buses were there not to collect fares, but to see that people got on the right bus for their destination, climbed the steps properly and got off at the right place, then many more incompetent people could travel around alone, go to work and enjoy a measure of independence and variety without fear of getting lost, assaulted or humiliated. Suppose there really was acceptable local collective child care, not just for the 'good' of the children, but also for that of the mothers?

The rise of medical institutions for the care and control of subnormal people in the nineteenth century has to be seen in the light of these considerations about labour requirements and family life. Clearly these are not the only considerations, and the role of alternative institutions such as pauper workhouses would also have to be taken into account.

What does the current trend away from medical domination of the field mean? It is very doubtful whether this trend towards greater educational control and more 'community' care represents a real change in the roles and status of subnormal people. It is well known that the projected 'community' care for the mentally ill and the dismantling of hospitals has hardly been the revolution it was supposed to be, nor has it happened to the extent proposed. There is every reason to suppose that the projected cut in subnormal patients in hospital (according to DHSS, 1971) to half their present number by 1991 will not happen in view of cutbacks in social service money. Further, the official emphasis on a more 'educational' approach to the subnormal, the new look which stresses how every individual should be given the opportunity to maximise his or her potential, has to be seen in terms of contemporary educational ideologies and goals. While physical conditions are likely to be better in schools and the new hostels than they are in the present hospitals, and while the staffing ratios and conditions of work may be improved (and with it the possibility of 'individual attention'), it is not the roles of the subnormal in society that will have changed, but merely the main institution of their enforcement.

This shift in the enforcement institutions from medicine to education is all part of the great upsurge of educational and psychological technology that has been increasingly used as a panacea for many social ills, for example the US anti-poverty 'Head Start' programmes. Certainly operant conditioning is extremely popular at the moment in the subnormal world (see below). The efficiency of educational institutions, and psychological technology, in performing the selection and training for a meritocratic society, while maintaining an ideology of equal opportunity, is undoubted. The 'purest' expression of this is in the notion of IQ that totally defines the subnormal, despite all attempts to introduce other criteria (see later). If anyone doubts how the philosophy of 'special' education for individual needs can be used against the supposed beneficiaries to confirm rather than change their social status, they should note that this is exactly the kind of philosophy that Jensen and others are espousing to deal with the 'social problem of familial and racial retardation'.

Leaving the question of the medical provision of care for the subnormal, let us turn to medical knowledge about the subnormal. Medical knowledge about mental subnormality mostly takes the form of description of syndromes and types, with attempted classifications according to either symptoms, or presumed causation and etiology, or both. Medical interest of this kind seems to have been virtually non-existent before the advent of institutions for the subnormal. Before about the 1870s stupidity was seen as a largely undifferentiated condition, with only cretins recognised somewhat earlier as a distinct subgroup, and only very occasional concern (for example Esquirol in France earlier in the century) with degrees of idiocy. The predominant concern seems to have been that of distinguishing the mad (dements) from the stupid (aments). Medical preoccupation with typologies was given a great impetus with Langdon-Down's description in 1866 of 'mongols' as a distinct group. Typologies then proliferated, such as Down's classification into congenital, development and accidental etiologies, and Ireland's twelve types. Modern medical textbooks (see, for example, Crome and Stern, 1967) abound with classifications and descriptions according to assumed cause or associated symptoms; and there are now a large number of recognised syndromes, especially extremely rare ones. One of the high points of medical research of this kind was the discovery of PKU (phenylketonuria) in 1934, and the subsequent analysis of its genetic and biochemical mechanisms, leading to one of the few curative treatments in the whole field. Incidentally, PKU is an extremely good example of how a 'genetic cause' of low intelligence does not mean that environmental manipulation is likely to be ineffective — exactly the reverse has been demonstrated. Another medical achievement of this kind has been the discovery of the chromasomal mechanisms involved in 'mongolism' in 1959. This however has not yet led to an understanding of what causes the chromasomal abnormalities, or to any effective treatment.

It seems widely agreed, even among doctors, that for a whole century's effort the results of this kind of approach to the causes and types of subnormality have been less than spectacular, especially when compared with the kind of progress made in medicine generally. Thus Richards (1970) says: 'Our ignorance of mental subnormality is such that a central theme of research... is still the preliminary one of attempting to segregate a large heterogeneous population into smaller homogeneous ones.' It is usually estimated that less than one-third of even the severely subnormal have a certain diagnosis, and that the majority of all the subnormal go unclassified. It is not surprising to find, therefore, that subnormality has an extremely low status within medicine. There are no spectacular careers or reputations to be made and much less money than in other branches of medicine. Doctors are given virtually no training in it (see Holt and Huntley, 1973, for the amount of time spent on the subject in medical schools), and their training in general does not fit them for dealing with a chronic condition for which there is no treatment, and where the sufferers are not really 'ill'.

Given how little medical care and medical knowledge have to offer those defined as subnormal, it becomes even more important to understand what medicine's functions have been and are, and how what has become known as the medical model has had such a great influence on other disciplines concerned with subnormality, to the virtual exclusion of any other approach.

## PSYCHOLOGY AND THE 'MEDICAL MODEL'

What is meant by 'the medical model'? First it should be said that by 'model' is not meant a precise theory or set of suggested mechanisms to explain an agreed range of phenomena, but something more general; a set of assumptions, ways of conceiving problems, a particular determination of what is held to be relevant and what not. Mercer (1973) provides a detailed account of what constitutes the medical model as regards subnormality, in contrast to a social system one. It should be noted that 'social' and 'medical' models are not necessarily in conflict with each other, because to some extent they actually are dealing with different problems. Conflicts do exist, however, especially as regards the supposed implications for educational philosophies, and research fund allocation. Further, one main argument is about the absence in medical and psychological approaches of *any* sociological perspectives at all, despite the lip service paid in introductory chapters of textbooks to the idea that medical subnormality is a social or cultural phenomenon. Medical categories of definition and diagnosis are seen as descriptive of pathological defects in the individual; the only social questions are those of the incidence and prevalence of defective individuals. While effort is put into the elaboration and refinement of instruments for the detection of defects, and their biological causes or associated conditions, very little attention is paid to the social and personal consequences of such categorisation. Indeed, the categorisation is not seen as an act that has any particular social meaning, except in terms of administrative decisions about future care or education. Just as the social roles and statuses of the people who are the object of categorisation are not seen as being of any relevance or interest, neither is the act of categorisation, or the statuses and roles of the people who carry it out or who deal with the products of such categorisation.

In what follows I shall consider some aspects of psychology that exemplify this 'medical' approach, in terms of the concepts, the techniques and the theories that psychology has introduced, and also in terms of the everyday activities of psychologists in medical and educational institutions. This account cannot be a comprehensive review of all the aspects of psychology, but it includes the most salient ones, namely *diagnosis*, definition and assessments; the IQ test and related notions of development; *typologising* of subnormals into different behavioural categories; *defect theories* of how subnormals differ from normals; and finally, the psychology of behavioural change — *operant conditioning* as one answer to the evils of institutions.

*Diagnosis*

Historically, psychology made its entry into the subnormality field with the invention of the intelligence tests. Before this no very certain means of diagnosis existed, though by the end of the nineteenth century there was increasing debate among doctors about the criteria to be used. Binet and Simon developed their test in response to a request from the Paris education authorities to provide a reliable method of identifying those dull children who would not benefit from education in the existing school system. The intelligence test was thus invented as a *diagnostic* instrument. Further, the ideas of relative mental age and of educability were introduced together, an association that has had important implications for subsequent debates on individual potential and educational equality of opportunity. The IQ test was accepted by medical and educational authorities in many countries as putting the diagnosis of stupidity on a 'scientific' basis. As well as allowing doctors to feel more confident in their diagnoses, it introduced the idea of a single continuum of intelligence, to the exclusion of all other notions. It also led to the 'discovery' of many more subnormals than had been thought existed, and contributed greatly to the eugenic scare of the period. That this was hailed as one of the achievements of IQ tests shows the value put on ascertainment, and especially on the assumption that ascertainment is without question a justifiable activity. Ascertainment is usually justified in terms of the need to provide services — the adverse consequences for those so ascertained is never part of the balance sheet. Mercer (1973) presents data showing that a substantial part of her sample would have been better off in terms of lessened stigma and discrimination, and certainly no worse off in terms of services, if they had never been diagnosed at all.

Along with the identification of increased numbers of subnormals, particularly 'higher-grade' ones, came disputes about where to draw the dividing line with normality: should it be IQ 70, 75, 80 or where? This demarcation dispute was, and still is, carried on as though it had some substance to it, and was not just a matter of statistical and administrative decision.

IQ tests and other related means of assessments have provided the major roles for clinical and educational psychologists. Recently there seems to have been growing dissatisfaction with this role and a search for other roles, with the suggestion that most assessment could safely be left to trained psychological technicians (Mittler, 1973). The role of clinical psychologists in subnormality hospitals seems to have been a particularly uncertain one — it is certainly a low-status one in the eyes of both other clinical psychologists and doctors. This is partly because it has never been very clear what psychologists in hospitals could offer, once the patients had been diagnosed, assessed and placed in high-, low- or other-grade wards, recommended for or excluded from occupational therapy or school. Until recently the number of psychologists has always been quite small, but their gradual increase seems to have been accompanied by increasing role uncertainty and dissatisfaction. Gunzberg (1973), in a review of the role of hospital psychologists, apart from a plea for greater humanity, suggests that psychologists should act as liaison officers between different disciplines and administrative departments, concerned with the management of overall life of the patient. This is hardly what clinical training is currently designed for.

It is interesting to ask why psychologists should now be becoming increasingly dissatisfied with their functions of diagnosis, assessment and selection, and not wish any longer to be seen as 'test bashers'. Perhaps this is due to the greater social criticism that has been directed at the IQ test as the instrument of educational selection and streaming, or perhaps to the increasing influence of various behavioural change ideologies that are currently seen as the main alternative approach to assessment (see Mittler, 1973). Or perhaps the professional status of psychology is changing in relevant ways.

The invention of intelligence tests has had a profound influence on the way in which psychologists have thought about subnormals, quite apart from providing them with diagnostic roles. The model of child development implicit in the concept of IQ is completely atheoretical as regards the process of development, about what constitutes change and how it happens. The different 'stages' are defined statistically, the content of the stages being determined more by the desired statistical properties of the resulting test than by any consideration of what is developmentally meaningful. Change is conceptualised as a series of quantitative accretions, not related in any particular way to the preceding or succeeding ones. Development is a competitive race up a single continuum of average scores. In most psychological research subnormals are defined only in terms of IQ, MA (mental age) and CA (chronological age). The individuals so specified are not allowed any other existence, social or biological, and the questions asked about subnormals are conceived only in terms of these parameters.

One of the major forms of psychological experiments has been to compare groups of different IQ (low and average) to see if they differ in certain respects — and it is held to be a serious problem of research strategy and methodology whether to match the different IQ groups in terms of MA or CA (see Ellis, 1963, 1969, for example). That no other variables are included in the model has lead to work that is grotesquely useless by *any* standards, for example, comparing institutionalised subnormals with normal children living at home, with no mention of social class or race. O'Connor and Hermelin (1963), much respected for the stringency and sophistication of their experimental designs, are a striking example of this howler. Such an absence of control is difficult to comprehend — given the obsession with control of other experimental variables, and the extensive data on the effects of institutionalisation on children — except in terms of the exclusion of all explicit social reference and meaning in the IQ model of development and the IQ tests themselves, and the psychologists' assumption that such abstraction of 'cognitive' abilities from social determinants is possible. A further explanation of why some of the psychology of subnormality has been so bad, even within its own terms of experimental matching and control, is because of the low level of competence of many of the psychologists in the field. The general stigma of subnormality rubs off on all the professions associated with it, and the whole topic of low intelligence has not attracted any outstanding psychologists. Again, there are no spectacular careers to be made in this branch of academic research.

There have been sporadic attempts to lessen the grip of the IQ definition of subnormals, but with little success. In the various textbooks and in the American Association on Mental Deficiency (AAMD) system of classification adopted in 1959, there is explicit acknowledgement that intellectual incompetence as measured by IQ is only one aspect of the inability to adapt, and that other criteria, especially pertaining to social skills, should be introduced as well. The use of social quotient, SQ, as judged by various tests is often advocated. However a study of institution records by Adams (1973) found that even with SQs available the IQ was overwhelmingly used by both doctors and psychologists in their evaluations and recommendations. Although one may well question both the kinds of tests that are used for 'social adaptiveness' and the values inherent in them, the use of other criteria has the advantage of showing up the particular and often covert social biases of the IQ test. Thus Mercer (1973) shows how many children classified and treated as subnormal on IQ criteria alone 'pass' other tests for social adaptiveness. Ethnic group and socioeconomic status were found to account for much more of the variance in IQ (15—20 per cent) than in 'adaptive behaviour' (almost none). The adaptive behaviour criteria covered a wide variety of social functions, including educational and occupational roles. Such criteria gave the same prevalence rates for Anglo or Caucasian subnormals as did the IQ test criterion, but greatly reduced the rates for Mexican-Americans and blacks, and a similar effect was found for socioeconomic status.

Mercer's findings illustrate the social and cultural biases inherent in a clinical approach, using traditional diagnostic criteria, leading to the 'ascertainment' of many people as subnormal who in fact were functioning quite unexceptionally in their own everyday social setting. Mercer's work also illustrates more convincingly than all previous work the way in which IQ tests are used as instruments of social discrimination under the guise of scientific neutrality. Existing medical and psychological practice in the field of subnormality, with its reliance on such normative scales, cannot assimilate these social implications because it does not have a framework for looking at its own social existence and status.

## Typologies

If medicine has used psychology to provide 'efficient' means of diagnosis for stupidity, and has thereby influenced most psychological work in the field, psychology has adopted medical mythology when it comes to describing and categorising subnormals. Using the model of classifying by a combination of apparent behaviour or symptoms, and presumed etiology, subnormals are categorised into two main types: 'organic' *v.* 'cultural — familial' in American terminology and 'pathological' *v.* 'subcultural' in English. This latter distinction was in fact first invented by an English doctor, Lewis, when asked to survey defective people for the Wood Commission in 1929. The etiological basis of the classification was the supposed source of variation in intelligence, normal sources of variation being distinguished from pathological ones. The behavioural basis was that the 'subcultural' group were supposed to be relatively high grade, of low socioeconomic status, with high family incidence of subnormality but with none of the physiological impairments allegedly found in the pathological group. The latter group tended to be lower grade intellectually, but with a more typical social class distribution.

This dichotomous classification is reproduced in many contemporary psychological textbooks, and widely used by many different authors (e.g. Clarke and Clarke, 1958; Penrose, 1963; Robinson and Robinson, 1965; Clausen, 1966; Zigler, 1967; Jensen, 1970). At its crudest it is an attempt to draw a distinction between 'biological' and 'social' cases, between those whose stupidity is due to biological mechanisms going wrong, and those whose stupidity is due to bad environment combined with poor quality but not abnormal genes — in short, the cycle of poverty and deprivation at the tail end of the normal distribution of intelligence. How truly 'social' the 'social' cases are regarded depends on whether you subscribe to the whole nature/nurture dichotomy and where in the percentage stakes you rate the 'inheritance' of difference in intelligence. Even those such as Jensen (1970) who rate it very high still persist in distinguishing between the two kinds of mechanisms of the production of intelligence, as also do those who take the most explicitly sociogenic perspectives. Mercer (1973), for example, identifies a 'hard-core' biological group. This dichotomy continues to be forced on the whole field despite the evidence and arguments that seriously query both its etiological basis and its empirical and behavioural significance. A brief outline of the case against this dichotomy is given here; a fuller one is found elsewhere (Ryan, 1971).

The distinction between pathological and normal sources of variation in intelligence is at best blurred and at worst unidentifiable. Our knowledge of the determinants of intelligence at any level is incomplete and gross, and it is clear that a multiple and complex interaction of a great many factors is involved. We have not even begun to conceptualise this interaction, let alone to measure it. We certainly do not know what 'causes' variation in intelligence within the statistically defined normal range, although we have collected many correlates of this variation. So the distinction between normal and pathological variation begs several all-important questions. Further, although reliable associations have been established between certain biological phenomena and low IQs in some cases, as in 'mongolism', there is still very great variation within these conditions. Thus in 'mongolism' the variation in recorded IQ is at least equal to four standard deviations (Penrose and Smith, 1966) and in PKU it is even greater, with many undiagnosed cases in the 'normal' range (Hsia, 1967). In other cases, such as maternal rubella, hydrocephalus and microcephaly, the association between these factors or conditions and low IQ is even grosser, and much less reliable. Many of the factors that covary with IQ within the normal range, such as education and social class, contribute to this variation within the subnormal range and in pathological cases. It also cannot be assumed that the genetic equipment of the individual, however that is specified, ceases to operate in the presence of other biological factors, though we know as little about this interaction as we do in 'normal' cases. Further, many people with IQs in the normal range have biological abnormalities, minor chromosomal damage, hydrocephalic conditions and biochemical 'errors', which if associated with low IQ would lead them to be classified as biological cases of stupidity. Are they 'biological cases' of normality? Are the rest of us 'social cases'?

Apart from its extremely weak theoretical basis, the dichotomy is always open to the finding that apparently 'social' cases of subnormality in fact have unsuspected biological involvements or consequences. For example poverty, ill health, inadequate diet, poor or non-existent perinatal care are all found frequently in the environment of the subcultural subnormals. It is implausible to suppose that these do not have direct biological effects which would be found if research workers or doctors were concerned to look for them. Birch *et al.* (1967) for example, found that more than half of an unselected sample of high-grade subnormal children, many of whom would be categorised as 'subcultural', had some kind of central nervous system dysfunctioning.

The dichotomy between cultural—familial and organic subnormals has no basis in empirical findings, in that no consistent differences have been found between the two groups despite extensive investigations (see Clausen, 1966, for a review of this evidence). Neither has any notable homogeneity in behaviour been found within either of the groups, which is not surprising considering the diversity involved. It is worth emphasising how much money, time and effort has gone into this attempt to find behavioural differences between the groups, because it is a comment both on research priorities of the time — categorisation — and on the investment in the validity of this distinction. Why is this dichotomy still propounded as a fact of subnormal life?

One possible explanation invokes the conceptual framework of medicine that psychology has adopted, namely the need to identify and classify those that medicine can deal with — the biological cases — and the acceptance of the nature/nurture dichotomy, and the crude causal models that go with this. While relevant, this is hardly an explanation.

Another explanation, not usually considered, is that the

distinction serves the interests of those who do most to maintain it. Subcultural subnormality is exclusively, and by definition, a lower social class and ethnic minority phenomenon. The middle classes and whites are represented, usually proportionate to their numbers at large, almost solely in the lower IQ and organic groups. A study of parents' organisations for the mentally retarded in the United States (Farber, 1968) shows that they are largely run by middle-class whites, for the benefit of their children. Lower social class and black parents of low IQ children, many with biological diagnoses, participate much less in these organisations. Further, there are many fewer such organisations for higher-grade children. Parents' organisations, among other things, collect money for research, and of course all research workers and professional workers are of middle-class and upper socioeconomic status, and tend to be white.

Subcultural subnormality has always been associated with a range of social evils — degeneration of the race, poverty, crime, promiscuity, cultural 'deprivation' — and there have always been demands for negative eugenics on these grounds. Middle-class families can escape some of this social stigma by identifying their stupid children as clearly different from the mass of lower social class stupid children. The identification of a biological 'accident' in a child can serve to remove the stigma of bad inheritance or bad environment and certainly remove the need for eugenic measures, since biological 'accidents' can rarely reproduce, or if they can the defect is not always transferable. (PKU is an exception here.) As mentioned above, there is a concentration of research resources in identifying many of the extremely rare biological causes of low-grade subnormality, and a neglect of possibly biological factors in subcultural subnormality. None of this is to deny the biological reality of such cases, or the usefulness of at least some of this knowledge, but to ask in whose interests it is, first to maintain a distinction between pathological and normal sources of variation in intelligence, and second, to spend, as a priority, a lot of money on identifying the rarer biological causes or conditions of low-grade subnormality and not do the same for the mass of lower social class and ethnic minority subnormals?

Apart from the pathological—subcultural classification, many other pseudo-biological ones have been proposed by psychologists, but those such as exogenous *v.* endogenous and primary *v.* secondary have gained less credence. The AAMD produced an intricate system of classification in 1959, based largely on presumed cause, which is not widely used. Strictly medical categories are increasingly being used in psychological research, and 'mongols' particularly are the target of efforts to establish brain-behaviour relationships.

## Defect theories

Defect theories proliferated during the last twenty years but are now less fashionable. They epitomise the influence of the medico-pathological model on psychology, carried to lengths that have precluded almost all other psychological approaches during this period. 'Defective' means part missing or not working, and the essence of these theories is that subnormals, over and above their slowness of development, are qualitatively different from 'normals' in that they also have specific impairments in particular functions. Most of these theories have only been concerned with cognitive development and functioning. They differ in the kind of specific defect postulated, but a great variety has been proposed (see Zigler, 1967, for a survey of such theories). Among such special defects are language and speech, short-term memory, attention and verbal encoding.

Defect theories are basically comparative theories, in that the alleged defect is identified relative to what is considered normal functioning. The comparison is always to the disadvantage, never to the advantage, of the subnormal. The basis of the comparison, and the methods used to establish the presence or absence of a defect, is of course the IQ model of development. Most defect theories equate subnormal and normal groups for stage of development and then compare them on the chosen aspect of behaviour. Mental age, as ascertained by an IQ test, is the indicator of equivalent development. The only notable defect theorist to use chronological age is Ellis (1963, 1969). Criticism of this comparative method and choice of mental age matching are only just beginning to be made, and psychologists have been loath to interpret their results or lack of them in terms of the methods used to set up their experiments. This is an example of what was referred to earlier, namely the total definition of subnormals for the purposes of psychological experiments in IQ terms.

The results of all this effort to identify defects have been very unsuccessful, even within the terms of reference of the psychologists in question. It has not proved possible to make many empirical generalisations about subnormal—normal differences, and the field is beset by conflicting or inconsistent findings. One further feature of this work is that subnormals are almost always found to be inferior to, or much less often equal to, the comparison groups of normals. There are virtually no findings of subnormal superiority. Given the allegedly equal basis of the matching methods used, one would not have expected this. This calls into question the context of these matching methods, the kinds of questions asked and the experimental methods used to answer them. All these are loaded against subnormals in various ways. The emphasis is entirely on what subnormals can't do, or can't do as well as normals, on defects or at best on the absence of defects — never on what they can or might do.

One of the assumptions behind defect theories is that some kind of organic impairment causes the defect, with no other kind of cause even theoretically being considered. The terms of reference here, as in many other parts of psychology, are entirely brain-behaviour ones. The problems arise within this framework when no neurological mechanisms or actual brain pathologies can be identified for correlation with observed behaviour. This is overwhelmingly the case with subnormals, since neurological and brain research is, compared with other more prestigious fields, very undeveloped, and because what knowledge there is does not lend itself to interpretation in terms of specific defects, but mostly concerns gross and diffuse pathologies. This absence of any actual physiological data, of the kind that is available in brain lesion work with adults or animals, has not stopped psychologists looking for this kind of explanation, or postulating theories that assume certain kinds of mythical brain mechanisms as reality. This again illustrates the strength of the medico-pathological model, in face of its evident lack of substantiation in its own terms or validation from empirical findings. Psychologists have filled the gap created by the absence of any hard physiological knowledge with their own peculiar ontology — fictional brain mechanisms. This activity, known as neurologising, was made respectable by Hebb in 1949, but was just about going out of fashion in general psychology when it caught on in the subnormality field — another example of the low-status phenomenon. Thus Ellis (1969) proposes 'inadequate stimulus trace strength' as the underlying defect.

A link is often made between the assumptions of defect theories and the organic—cultural familial typology discussed above. Thus the Clarkes (1973b) find the defect position 'tempting' on the grounds that a large number of subnormals have organic impairments, despite acknowledging the negative behavioural evidence for the typology. Zigler (1967) maintains that defect approaches should be confined to those known to have some organic impairment, and he proposes a different model for the allegedly non-organic cases. This is known as the developmental model, in which the subnormals in question are seen as developing essentially normally, only much more slowly, but suffering from all the adverse consequences of slow development and categorisation as subnormal — frequent failure, lack of self-reliance, fear of more failure, and institutionalisation. These social and motivational consequences of labelled subnormality are held to affect an individual's cognitive functioning in certain usually detrimental ways, and Zigler tries to explain the differences he finds between normals and these subnormals in terms of the ensuing cognitive strategies. While this kind of approach is a welcome breath of social reality in a field dominated by pathological superstition, it has not really been pursued very far by other psychologists and has met with a lot of heated opposition from Ellis (1969) and others.

The main problem with Zigler's approach is that its rationale lies in the distinction between 'organic' and 'cultural—familial' subnormality. He does not extend his model to those he considers definitely to have a hole in the head. Indeed, his justification for his model depends on being able to distinguish these cases. While arguing for a more 'socially' orientated approach to some subnormals, he relegates to the pathological model the superficially more plausible cases, quite forgetting that they too have a social existence, and thus reinforces the typology. Other theorists who argue even more strongly than Zigler for a 'social' approach to subnormals also fall into this trap of excluding what are felt to be the clearly biological cases from their models. Thus Mercer (1973), for all her argument against an exclusively medical model, is content at the end of her book to distinguish individuals according to whether they are biologically impaired or not.

*Operant conditioning*

A short consideration of this is relevant here, not because it is an instance of the medico-pathological influence in psychology, but because it appears to be replacing this influence, to some extent. The philosophy of this brand of behaviourism in fact eschews any speculation or theory about what is going on inside an organism, and in most of its approaches does not appear interested in the 'causes' of subnormality, with the exception of Bijou's (1967) attempt to see the production of subnormality entirely in terms of the wrong reinforcement schedules. Operant conditioning, though it focuses on the immediate environmental control of behaviour, cannot be said to represent a genuinely 'social' approach, because of its extremely narrow and mechanical conception of what the environment is for any individual. 'The environment' does not extend much beyond the dispensation of food and praise, punishment and disapproval. Who the dispensers of reinforcement are, how they got into these roles, why the receivers are the people they are, what the institutions, expectations, power relations and categories of thought are that have thrown and kept the two together, is out of bounds for this approach. Operant conditioning has thus become an adjunct to and not a threat to the prevailing conceptions and institutions of subnormality. It has also allowed psychologists a new lease of life, which even they were beginning to realise they needed (see Clarke and Clarke, 1973a, and Mittler, 1973, for a discussion of this).

To date the most extensive applications of operant conditioning techniques have been in the back wards of hospitals where the most serious problems of management, and the worst conditions, occur. In many programmes the undesirable behaviour of the patients is carefully defined, and the nurses are trained by psychologists in techniques for the elimination of this and the substitution of more desirable 'responses'. Such programmes in the main do nothing to change the institutional structure or physical conditions of hospital wards — indeed, they make the running of such wards smoother. The behavioural problem to be managed is still located in the individual subnormal, just as his defect was. Psychology has once again been enlisted as a managerial prop to a prevailing institutional need.

Operant conditioning provides a more efficient means of control over an individual's behaviour than any that education or psychology has provided so far (see Ryan, 1975, for a more detailed consideration of this). It is no coincidence that the administrative transfer of the training centres and schools from medicine to education comes at a time of increasingly efficient educational technology. The ideology of 'better services for the mentally handicapped' (DHSS, 1971) — that each individual should have his or her potential maximised through appropriate training — requires the justification for the idea of potential and the technology for measuring it — IQ tests — as well as the technology for realising it in a sufficiently flexible way to meet individual differences — behaviour modification.

CONCLUSION

This chapter presents a preliminary account of the extremely complex question of how the kind of psychology that is done, both 'pure' and 'applied', reflects and reinforces some implicit ideological assumptions concerning the place of the inept in our society. The various activities of psychologists — diagnosis, assessment, research, behaviour modification — all have a particular relation to the social processes that create and maintain so many people as 'stupid'. The purpose of this chapter has been not to adopt the artificial dichotomy between the biological and the social, nor to weigh in more heavily on the side of the social. Neither has there been any attempt to deny the operation — real as opposed to mythical — of biological factors. Rather, the aim has been to demonstrate how psychology's exclusive concern with biological and pathological 'explanations' is in itself a reflection of the social and political system that has produced so many marginal people, and also so many psychologists to deal with them. The problem is always located in 'them' and never in 'us' — 'we' only care and help and objectively investigate. If 'they' do not respond or improve as much as 'we' hope, this is because of the inherent hopelessness of 'them', and nothing to do with the society that has created 'us', 'them' and our relationships with each other. Psychology, in its adoption of medical model thinking and practice, has created a pseudo-science that prevents any consideration of the social existence either of those it categorises or of psychologists themselves. In so doing it exacerbates the problem it is allegedly trying to alleviate.

## NOTES

1 A note on terminology — the descriptive terms used in this field change with great rapidity in the fruitless search for value-free labels. Here, 'idiocy', 'stupidity', 'mental deficiency', 'subnormality' and 'mental retardation' are used interchangeably as the context merits. The more euphemistic ones (e.g. 'exceptionality') are avoided.

# 11 Psychiatry and the Medical Mandate

## by Nigel Goldie

In recent years the involvement of the medical profession in the treatment of 'mental illness' and other forms of deviant behaviour has been increasingly questioned and criticised. Such criticisms have come from various directions, psychiatrists themselves often being the most forthright critics of the activities of their colleagues (e.g. Laing, 1960; Cooper, 1967; Szasz, 1970). To many psychiatrists, however, the 1959 Mental Health Act and the powers that it entrusted to them, and more recently the decision to establish psychiatric units in general hospitals, have been taken as evidence of society's recognition of their claims to be *the* profession to control the treatment and care of the mentally ill (Hill, 1969). While such developments appear to have strengthened the institutional position of psychiatry, the emergence and growth of other occupations also laying claim to being able to treat mental patients poses certain problems for psychiatric practitioners. Psychiatrists have frequently been regarded as 'marginal' medical men. But if they are marginal in relation to the rest of medicine, they are also marginal in their relations to other disciplines and occupations. There have been several studies in the United States of the problems that psychiatrists, especially beginners, encounter in their relations with other staff (see Martin, 1962; Sharaf and Levinson, 1964; Smith, 1957). They have undergone the same medical training and socialisation experience as other medical specialists, but the skills and techniques that they use in their daily working lives are more likely to be those of the social workers, nurses and clinical psychologists, rather than those taught in their medical schools. Further, the organisational procedures and working practices of most mental hospitals, whether 'therapeutic communities' or not, invariably involves the psychiatrist in working in a 'team' with members of other occupations, who may claim to have as great if not greater expertise at treating and handling mental patients. As Goffman (1968) has pointed out:

> Professional psychiatric staff itself does not have an easy role. The members' medical licence gives them one of the firmest claims to deference and regard available in our society, and one of the firmest expert service occupations, yet in the mental hospital their whole role is constantly in question. Everything that goes on in the hospital must be legitimated by assimilating it or translating it to fit into a medical-service frame of reference. [p. 334]

If it is assumed that such occupations as psychiatric social work and clinical psychology are making an implicit, if not particularly open, challenge to psychiatrists, the problem then becomes one of accounting for the continued dominance of psychiatry over other occupations. The answer to this question cannot be found through a theory of 'technical determinism'; the medical profession had established control over the institutional 'treatment' of patients long before they possessed any efficacious techniques or therapies. The continuing controversy over the lasting therapeutic value of present-day physical treatment undermines those claims that there are proven mechanistic and technical means available to psychiatrists, even if such treatments are relied upon for administrative and other reasons. One approach to developing an understanding of the ways in which an established and powerful occupation is able to maintain its dominance over possible rivals would be through social historical analysis of the origins of that profession, and in particular of its relations with other powerful interests. However, the concern of this book is with 'everyday medical life', and thus the focus of this chapter is on one aspect of the way the dominance of psychiatrists, over the treatment of mental illness, is sustained and legitimised in daily practice. The aim is to explore the nature of the ideology held by a group of psychiatrists, which gives expression to the way that they seek to legitimise their control over the treatment of mental illness.

In recent years increasing attention has been given to the way in which emergent factions, segments and divisions within and between occupations can be identified through an analysis of the ideologies to be found among their members (Schatzman and Strauss, 1966).

Atkinson, Reid and Sheldrake (1972) have noted how:

> Such ideologies are not arbitrary but rather are articulated around a set of important dimensions, one of the most important of which is indeterminacy / technicality; others that are important include superiority/inferiority and autonomy and dependance. Running through these ideologies and linking the particular points on the various dimensions that characterise them is the notion of control, and it is control that we see as the touchstone to understanding professional process. [pp. 14—15]

'Technicality / indeterminacy' refers to the work of Jamous and Peliolle (1970), who have argued that occupations or factions within occupations that claim to possess technical skills have tended to usurp control from those who claim that their skills reside in their indeterminate and private or personal, knowledge and abilities. Perhaps more clearly than within any other branch of medicine, there have been conflicts among psychiatrists over the technical as opposed to indeterminate nature of their skills. Thus in any consideration of the relationship of psychiatrists to other occupations, it is important to identify the nature of the expertise that psychiatrists claim to possess, and the consequences of such claims for possible rivals.

At the present time psychiatrists are largely able to define the terms on which the members of such aspiring professions as psychiatric social work and clinical psychology have access to patients. Psychiatrists are the key 'audiences' for these occupations, and their expectations and regard for them to a certain extent determine how far they are able to 'professionalise', that is to gain control over the application of those skills and knowledge that they claim to be their own.

The concern of this chapter is thus with what has been termed 'the medical mandate', that is with the ideology that serves to sustain the control of psychiatrists over the treatment of mental illness. The 'medical mandate' is taken to comprise a series of interrelated assumptions and beliefs that provide rationales for the claim that mental illness is a primarily medical problem, even though it is also recognised as being more than that.

Secondly, there is the claim that psychiatry, as it is presently constituted, makes an essential contribution to the treatment of mental illness, the importance of this assumption being the supremacy claimed for psychiatric knowledge over other knowledge.

Thirdly, and strategically most important of all, there is the claim that there should be medical hegemony or leadership over other staff.

Finally, there are various claims made about psychiatric expertise and the extent to which both technical and indeterminate skill are held to be the basis of the psychiatrists' 'superior clinical judgement'. Beyond this there will be an attempt to illustrate the consequences of this mandate, through an analysis of the psychiatrists' attitudes towards the lay staff.

The material that is presented in this chapter is drawn from interviews with thirty-eight psychiatrists working in three large mental hospitals. One of the hospitals has a national reputation for its development of the 'therapeutic community' approach; another was run according to more traditional lines; while the third was a subnormality hospital. The interviews with the thirty-eight psychiatrists were structured in so far as a series of questions was asked of each psychiatrist. However, these were all open-ended questions and as far as possible the interviews took the form of conversations. During the field work stage that involved periods of non-participant observations, and subsequently during the analysis of the interviews, certain important differences of outlook among psychiatrists became apparent.

Other studies have drawn attention to the fragmented nature of the psychiatric profession. They have stressed conflicting attitudes towards the treatment of mental patients and the etiology of mental illness (Goldie, 1974; Marx, 1969). However, in the present study, the main differences appeared to be more over the psychiatrists' differing conceptions of their own role and their expectations of the other staff, than over their attitudes towards treatment. Three different types of psychiatrist were identified and these have been termed 'doctors' (of which there were 17), 'eclectics' (19) and 'dissidents' (2). Before considering the nature of the 'medical mandate' it is necessary to note the main differences between the two predominant groups, as there will be further references to them throughout the chapter.

As the term 'doctor' implies, such psychiatrists tended to present themselves as 'medical practitioners' or 'physicians', and some even doubted the value of having a separate specialty of psychiatry. Such psychiatrists stress the importance of medical knowledge and believe it to be crucial when deciding the diagnosis and treatment of patients. These activities are held to be the core activities of the psychiatrists, and in this sense a 'restricted' view of their own expertise is held. As might be expected, such psychiatrists favour 'medical' treatments, but are not necessarily opposed to other forms of treatment. Indeed, most of them assume that they can carry them out if they thought they were necessary. In line with their belief that their role was the same as any other doctor's, such psychiatrists believe they should direct the activities of other staff, and while the lay staff might make a useful contribution it must nevertheless be an auxiliary one to their own. In their eyes there need be no overlap or confusion over who does what, as long as everyone carries out those activities for which they have been trained.

By way of contrast, the 'eclectic' psychiatrists were those who believe that they can contribute to all aspects of the patients' situation. Thus they believe themselves to be aware not only of the medical but also of the social and psychological factors affecting the patients. Consequently they are more likely to talk of social workers and psychologists making an 'equal' contribution, and of claiming to 'let them contribute in whatever way they like'. Such psychiatrists tend to hold essentially 'liberal' and 'voluntaristic' philosophies, according to which they believe they are not directing the other staff, but merely offering 'guidance' or acting as a co-ordinator. Indeed, such activities are more likely to be claimed as the essential task of a psychiatrist rather than the actual treating of patients. Claiming to be eclectic in their attitude towards treatment, such psychiatrists generally accept the need for physical treatment, while suggesting that some form of psychotherapy will be more effective in the long run.

The dissident mode of response was more common among the social workers and psychologists, and thus it is not being given much attention in this chapter. Basically, they tended to support the 'anti-psychiatry' position and to be much more critical than their colleagues of the medical model and the structure and function of the mental health services. A detailed analysis of the 'dissident' mode of response and of other ideologies among social workers and clinical psychologists is to be found elsewhere (Goldie, 1974).

MENTAL ILLNESS AS A MEDICAL PROBLEM

As might be expected, a majority (twenty-nine) of the psychiatrists who were interviewed stated that they thought of mental illness as a medical problem, while the remainder were somewhat equivocal. Among the former there were several who suggested that it was 'more than a medical problem', but also others who simply asserted: 'It is and should be a medical problem' without going into more detail. In other words, some psychiatrists appeared to consider that no more need be said to such a question. Others, however, provided a variety of rationales or justifications for this belief. Several, for example, sought justification by referring to such 'technical' considerations as diagnosis:

> It has to be in the hands of the medical profession because of the problems of diagnosis. So many problems are caused by physical illness and organic conditions, that this side must be kept continually in mind. . . . It is absolutely essential for a psychiatrist to be a good physician, to have one's membership of the Royal College of Physicians. The more extensive your knowledge of medicine the better, there should be no question of psychiatrists being anything other than doctors.   [303]

(The first figure given in the coding numbers refers to the setting — thus the figure 1 refers to the 'therapeutic community' hospital, 2 to the more 'conventional' hospital and 3 to the subnormality hospital. The latter two figures identify the individual psychiatrist.)

This quotation echoes many of the features of the 'doctor' mode of response that has already been briefly described. In particular, the emphasis upon the importance of medical knowledge and the blanket assertion that mental illness is likely to be physical in origin provide a justification for psychiatry in traditional medical terms. As one stated, 'It is an illness like cancer is an illness.' Others were less assertive and talked of the *possibility* of there being a physical illness. As one of them said, 'Some psychiatric illnesses are associated with physical illness, such as dementia with pneumonia, and are therefore a medical problem in that sense' (120). Others raised further medical considerations, such as the evaluation of the side effects of drugs, or such routine problems as: 'If there were no doctors then the patients would have to be sent for routine physical examinations.

This would be time-consuming and expensive and besides nobody would want the job. Also I do not think that lay people can take over responsibility for the administration of drugs' (107).

Some of the 'doctors' who asserted that mental illness was a medical problem also referred to the administration of drugs as the crucial consideration: 'It has to be a medical problem because of the problem of the psychoses. If you treat psychotic illnesses you have to use drugs, and we are the only people who know about them' (205). While most of those who were sure that mental illness was a medical problem justified their position by reference to specific problems like those mentioned above, there were others who made very general and holistic claims. One psychiatrist for example claimed that:

> You cannot differentiate between mind and body. If the person is anxious his body is affected — they are interrelated. All psychiatric illnesses affect the body, the body affects the mental condition. So psychiatric illness is a medical problem. People have called the mind a tissue, which makes it as much a medical problem as any organ of the body.   [112]

Such reasoning appeared frequently, and it expresses clearly some of the assumptions upon which many psychiatrists rest their belief that, by definition, anyone who is 'mentally ill' should be seen by a psychiatrist. One psychiatrist went so far as to claim that: 'Mentally ill people cannot be treated without psychiatry. Anyone who is diagnosed as suffering from a mental illness must be seen by a psychiatrist . . . psychiatry is a medical speciality, so obviously he is the one to deal with mental illness' (304).

Other psychiatrists were rather more equivocal and stressed how mental illness was more than a medical problem. They often raised the problem of where to draw the line, especially when considering the neuroses and the personality disorders. One of them pointed out how, while they could not cure such conditions, 'The assumption is at the moment that these are medical problems, but one must not be rigid about it. In the future some things may be split off, so they won't require a doctor. But the initial screening must always be done by a doctor to eliminate the medical conditions' (101).

The more 'liberal' and 'open-minded' attitudes of the 'eclectic' psychiatrists can be seen in comments such as: 'This is a question that has been decided for us by other people. They expect us to treat such patients. The boundaries of medicine are very diffuse, while the traditions of medicine are respected and trusted by the general public. It cannot work any other way' (113).

Thus, although there were some psychiatrists who talked of 'the limitation of the medical model', or the need to see mental illness also as a 'social problem', the majority were convinced that it was first and foremost a medical problem. The consequences of this belief can be seen in the following quotation:

> It should be [seen as a medical problem], though in practice it is society that has decided this, it's not one's own choice. With some conditions it can be otherwise, but for the care of the acutely ill and disturbed psychiatric patient, the doctor must have the final say. Whatever you see as causing mental illness, and there are some organic conditions, all people with psychiatric disturbances must be vetted by a doctor first. So in this stage the doctor must have the overall control as many of those conditions are not recognisable to someone without his training. Besides, large sections of mental illness can now be treated with physical methods, and you need a doctor for this. The introduction of the phenothiazines has been the greatest advance in the treatment of mental illness, even if we are only controlling certain mental states, rather than curing them. [106]

This quotation provides a good example of what is termed the 'medical mandate' being claimed by psychiatrists. Not only is there the claim that 'others' have put the psychiatrists into a position of leadership, but there is also the assumption that, because some psychiatric illnesses are organic in origin, then all patients must be vetted by a doctor first. Not that such vetting takes an advisory form only, but it is regarded as a preliminary to the prescribing of drugs which must be under the control of the medical profession. These drugs are further claimed to be efficacious as if this was beyond dispute. Beyond this, the legitimacy of the medical model is so taken for granted that it is only natural that the doctor should have the final say, as he would over the care of the physically ill. Above all, there is the assumption that it is the right of the doctor to extend his basic mandate to treat physical illness to all matters affecting the patient even when there is no physical illness present. Thus, such psychiatrists believe that they not only have a right to decide on the relevance of their own contribution, but also that of the other staff. This point will be discussed later in the chapter.

## PSYCHIATRY AS THE TREATMENT OF MENTAL ILLNESS

Most of the psychiatrists clearly believed psychiatry to be essential for the treatment of mental illness. Indeed, it would have been surprising for any psychiatrist to have denied the value of his own specialty. However, the question cannot be left there; for the justifications given for the assertion that psychiatry is essential provide further evidence of the pervasive and diffuse medical ideology that supports the position of psychiatry.

Like the psychiatrists who believed that mentally ill people cannot be treated without psychiatry, there were others who asserted that psychiatry, by definition, was the essence of *any* treatment. Others were more specific in asserting the primacy of physical factors in causing the disturbance:

> The illness itself will have some biological correlates and particularly with schizophrenics, manias and depressions may be primarily biological, stemming from a disturbance in the central nervous system. In so far as there is physical ill health, the patient needs to be treated on the medical model. To talk of mental illness being a myth is nonsense. Doctors have to be involved because many mental illnesses are physical in origins being neither environmentally caused nor functional.   [201]

Significantly, while some psychiatrists, like the one quoted above, considered schizophrenia to be an organic illness, there were others who saw it as being a functional one. For example:

> The psychiatrist has to decide all the time whether he is dealing with an organic or functional disorder. Schizophrenia, for example, is more likely to be functional, in which case other people can be involved. Even so, the overall care of the patient must remain with the doctors as a class. They have been trained for this, and this should not be in the hands of anyone else.   [102]

This reveals very clearly the belief that only psychiatrists can decide the diagnosis and, further, that they 'as a class' are the only people fitted to take on responsibilities for treatment. However, while some psychiatrists believe themselves to possess certain scientifically proven 'technical knowledge', there are others who stressed how indeterminate and uncertain their knowledge was:

Deciding the diagnosis is the most important thing of all. For this you need someone who is experienced with mentally ill patients. Psychiatry is such an inexact science that each patient has to be treated separately. Most patients need drugs and mental illness is so vast and complicated that there is a need for the doctor to draw together all the hands, and to act as a co-ordinator. To get other people to help you. The initial assessment is the most important thing that we do; we often go wrong — it's a terrible mixture of clinical experience, general knowledge, and intuitive judgement.    [203]

This psychiatrist was not alone in referring to 'intuitive judgement', as there were many others who also talked of having 'special understanding', 'all-round knowledge', 'clinical experience' or a 'special sense' that enabled them to understand mental patients better than the other staff. It was not, of course, simply a matter of some psychiatrists claiming to possess 'technical knowledge' and others claiming indeterminate, intuitive abilities, but rather that both rationales were invoked by the same psychiatrists. More importantly, however, there were claims made, as by (203) above, that the act of diagnosis must be an exclusively medical affair. In view of the strategic importance of diagnosis, this claim illustrated very clearly the way in which psychiatrists seek to maintain control over what happens to patients.

Although it is being suggested that psychiatrists seek to maintain their control over certain processes, there were a few psychiatrists who were critical of the present arrangements. For example, some of the more dissident psychiatrists considered they were only essential because of the need to use drugs to control the behaviour of patients, and that beyond that they had nothing special to contribute. Many others noted the limitations of physical treatments, while some thought they were only effective in conjunction with other forms of therapy.

Other psychiatrists, especially eclectics, suggested they were essential because they had legal responsibility for the patients. They often said that they did not believe they made a more important contribution than the other staff, but that 'other staff', 'the patients' or 'the general public' expected them to make a more important contribution.

## THE JUSTIFICATION FOR MEDICAL HEGEMONY

It has already been observed how the 'doctor' psychiatrists tend to assert the need for medical direction in psychiatry in the same way as in surgery or some other branch of medicine. As one said, 'It is vital that there is medical direction. It is important that there is a boss, this is something I feel very strongly about' (201). Another talked of how 'The hierarchy is always there, and I don't think that it is the aim of the therapeutic community to knock out the hierarchy. I cannot see anything working without the hierarchy — it reduces anxiety. So it is only natural that we have control over those beneath us' (113).

By contrast, one of the 'dissident' psychiatrists commented that: 'It is not at all necessary for there to be a medical direction, except that our society is conditioned to authoritarianism. Not only do doctors themselves want to have complete control — this is after all, what our training has brought us to believe is our natural right — but the other staff expect to be led' (115).

However, most psychiatrists reiterated certain commonplace assumptions such as, 'If the medical profession has legal responsibility, then it has to have some directive powers' (307), the implication being that this authority is not of one's own choosing, but rather something imposed upon one. Such claims were even more clearly articulated by the more eclectic psychiatrists. For example:

> The psychiatrists are members of the team, alongside the other members of the team. They are not necessarily the leaders of the team. One has a certain amount of formal authority, but the extent to which the doctor is the leader of the team is very much dependent upon what others think of this role. I don't think that hierarchical structures are a good thing, or that the doctor should necessarily be the leader . . . as it is, the psychiatrist is the leader in the community and we are important at keeping the team together and keeping a watchful eye over what is going on.  [120]

It was suggested above that some psychiatrists claim they are essential only because 'other' people make them so. In the above quotation there is the same suggestion that 'others' have decided that they should provide the leadership and that consequently they must fulfil, and live up to, the 'others'' expectations. At the same time there is the contradiction of claiming to be merely a member of the team, while 'keeping a watchful eye' on what is going on. As noted earlier, such psychiatrists usually attach particular significance to their 'leadership role', even if they did talk more frequently of providing 'guidance', 'co-ordination' or 'advice' instead of 'direction' or 'supervision', as the 'doctor' psychiatrists tended to do. Further, whereas the doctors saw their authority as an extension of their right and duty to treat physical illness, the eclectics, who often sought to dissociate themselves from this restricted view of their role, attempted to justify their superior position either by suggesting it was forced upon them by the wider society or by claiming that their all-round experience gave them a 'greater understanding' than that possessed by the other staff.

## THE PSYCHIATRISTS' VIEW OF THEIR OWN EXPERTISE

In the course of outlining the medical mandate, several quotations have been given that indicate the kind of claims that psychiatrists make when talking about their skills. Clearly there are some psychiatrists, particularly the 'doctors', who believe that their knowledge of physical medicine forms the basis of their expertise when treating mental patients. Some 'doctors' *limited* their expertise to such activities as giving physical treatments and the related activities; for example, 'No one else can administer pharmacological therapies, and these are absolutely essential with the psychoses. It doesn't matter who treats the neurotics' (109). Many other psychiatrists appeared to regard the administration of physical treatment, especially the giving of ECT, to be very routine and a generally unrewarding activity. Overall, there were very few psychiatrists who wished to be thought of as 'pill pushers', even though most of the psychiatrists noted how they had to rely on physical treatments.

Instead the majority of the psychiatrists described themselves as variously being, 'therapists', 'psychotherapists', 'administrators', 'teachers', 'researchers', 'culture carriers', 'team leaders', 'co-ordinators'. In other words, while some suggested that they had therapeutic skills that extended beyond prescribing pills, most of them mentioned tasks that can best be described as administrative. One talked of

. . . being more of an administrator than a psychiatrist. I see myself to be primarily a team energiser, which means basically co-ordinating the efforts of other staff, while at the same time trying to decide upon a policy for each team and ward. This should be done through discussion and persuasion, but at the same time the consultant has the ultimate responsibility for deciding the policy of the unit.   [302]

Another spoke of the way he extended his work beyond that of treating patients:

My role is not only with treating the patient, but also acting as a medical administrator. Further, I co-ordinate the team and am responsible for the patient. I work mostly as a co-ordinator, but I am also a consultant in the sense of being an adviser and teacher to the rest of the team. When dealing with out-patients, I am much more individually involved. I tend to do my own diagnostic work and to refer people on for psychotherapy. Sometimes I take on patients for psychotherapy myself, and I also supervise the therapy that the junior staff carry out.   [200]

Several other psychiatrists talked of their 'all-round understanding', of how they 'saw the patient's situation as a whole' or had to 'examine the total life situation of the patient', or in some other way suggested that they had a more complete understanding of the patient's situation than the other staff. Such claims were sometimes backed up with references to the way that psychiatrists 'had to know about sociology and psychology as well as medicine'.

According to Henry, Sims and Spray (1971), 'psychotherapy' would appear to be the activity that most American mental health staff claim to carry out. Such a finding may be culture-bound in view of the greater popularity of psychotherapy in the United States. Certainly very few of the study psychiatrists claimed to be psychotherapists. Although most of them said they could carry it out, hardly any of them appeared to have had any training at it. It was generally assumed that they could carry it out, or could supervise other staff carrying it out, in the same way as it was assumed that they had a right to administer ECT. Among the more eclectic psychiatrists, there was a tendency to suggest that 'psychotherapy' could provide the ony 'real' or 'effective' therapy. But as the term 'psychotherapy' can be used to refer to anything from depth psychoanalysis to ECT, such beliefs must be related to the meaning that is attached to it.

Returning to the importance attached to 'administrative duties', some psychiatrists attached particular emphasis to the admission and discharge of patients. These were seen as activities that only they could carry out. Some defended this in terms of the need for 'psychiatric' knowledge when making such decisions, whereas others sought justification by referring to the limitations of the 'current administrative practices', as if these could not be changed. Such decisions are of strategic importance for the fate of patients and for the opportunities for other staff to fulfil their own claimed mandates. The way in which most psychiatrists sought to convey the impression that such arrangements could not be otherwise, and further how they imbue administrative activities with a medical mystique, provides an example of the pervasiveness of the general medical ideology according to which 'only doctors' can make certain decisions.

Many more references were made to various administrative tasks being the essential prerogative of the psychiatrists than were made to treatment activities. This was especially so with the eclectic psychiatrists. As one observed,

> I have an overall function relating to the admission wards, that I would see as a sort of guidance role, to see that the staff are balanced and that the team is not consultant-dominated or medically oriented. One cannot escape from a good deal of responsibility without guiding the unit, but one must be careful not to become an authority figure.   [104]

By showing insight into one's own relationships with other staff, by warning against becoming an 'authority figure' and by generally presenting oneself as being non-directive, while at the same time noting in passing that one has 'responsibility', the attempt is made to legitimise one's position through an appeal to reasonableness.

THE PSYCHIATRISTS' VIEW OF THE LAY STAFF

Earlier this century when social workers and clinical psychologists were first being introduced into mental hospitals they frequently encountered resistance, if not outright opposition, from the medical profession. By way of contrast, it would be unusual today to find a psychiatrist who was totally opposed to social workers even though there are some who consider, as one psychiatrist did, that 'psychologists are a waste of the taxpayer's money and the sooner their fraud is discovered the better' (105). Among the study psychiatrists there was near universal recognition of the 'importance' of social work and frequent comments such as, 'If the social worker does not do her job properly then the whole thing breaks down', or 'We could not manage without one' (203). Comments such as these, though, cannot be taken in isolation from the reasons given for the social workers being seen to be 'essential'. Stated briefly and at the risk of over-simplification, most psychiatrists recognise that social workers can and should carry out a wide range of activities ranging from 'gathering information', 'interviewing relatives' and dealing with 'social and practical problems' to 'being supportive' to the patients and relatives, 'contacting employers', 'finding accommodation' and so on.

If psychiatric units are to achieve the currently desired turnover, it is essential that someone carries out these tasks. However, nearly all these largely 'welfare' activities are *supplementary* to the treatment being given by the psychiatrists rather than being integral to it. Some psychiatrists, especially the 'eclectics', might talk of how social workers can act as 'therapists' with patients or their families, but there will rarely be any suggestion that they have any greater theoretical understanding, or even practical ability, in such tasks. Indeed, they will generally detract from the ideas that such lay staff have superior skills to themselves by such statements as: 'In the actual treatment situation, the role is interchangeable. Anyone on the staff could support the patient or give supportive psychotherapy. It really does not matter who carries it out' (205).

Whereas social workers have become functionally indispensable to the smooth running of most psychiatric units, the same cannot be said for clinical psychologists. While most psychiatrists will acknowledge that psychologists can provide additional information on diagnostic problems, such information is nearly always treated as ancillary to their own knowledge. As one psychiatrist put it, 'I would never treat a patient simply on the word of a psychologist; such decisions must always be left in the hands of the doctors' (206). Thus psychologists are seen as 'path. lab assistants' even if it is acknowledged that they also teach and carry out research. Some psychiatrists, while recognising that psychologists can carry out therapy, and even deferring in some cases to the psychologists over the question of behaviour therapy, are usually quick to assert how psychologists are no better at psychotherapy than anyone else.

It would be a mistake to suggest that psychiatrists never acknowledge or suggest that lay staff have special abilities, but when they do it is nearly always for *particular* reasons. One of the 'eclectic' psychiatrists, for example, made the following observation about clinical psychologists:

> Their contribution is limited in psychiatric practice. Maybe it's because they have been trained wrongly, or maybe it's because we approach things from different angles. . . . I have known other hospitals where the psychologist was very involved with what went on in the admission unit. She could contribute by providing a slightly different approach. But this is a personality thing, for their training as psychologists doesn't appear to have much relevance for practising psychiatry.  [106]

Within this quotation there is the contradiction of on the one hand valuing the 'different approach' of the psychologists, and on the other attributing their lack of 'clinical relevance' to having precisely a 'different angle'. This contradiction is resolved by seeing it all in terms of personality, thereby negating any 'professional' contribution that clinical psychologists as a group might make.

As with social workers, it is assumed that the only criterion by which to judge the value of the psychologists' contribution is that of psychiatric practice. While it might be recognised that some lay staff make 'valuable' contributions, such recognition is nearly always granted to particular individuals who have the appropriate 'personality'. The criteria on which such assessments are made are rarely spelt out, the assumption being that the psychiatrist's all-round ability enables him to identify such talents; as one of them expressed it, 'I consider it is the task of the consultant to make the best of whatever is the best in each member . . . it is he who must mobilise resources. There is a need for leadership, and the doctor is the natural person to provide it. No one else can be as comprehensive as the doctor can be' (108).

Conclusion

Many British psychiatrists like to believe that they are 'non-ideological' in so far as they do not adhere or identify with any one particular school of thought, or for that matter hold strong and rigid views about their work. The aim of this chapter has been to suggest that many of the apparently 'commonsense' and 'taken-for-granted' assumptions that are frequently expressed by psychiatrists, such as those quoted above, are indeed ideological, and further that they provide rationales for defending current control of the medical profession over the institutionalised treatment of mental illness. Psychiatrists can always justify this control by referring to the 1959 Mental Health Act and the powers that it entrusted in them. But the majority appear to seek to legitimise their position either by referring to such 'rational' factors as the need for them to administer physical treatments, or by suggesting that there is a certain naturalness and inevitability about the present arrangements. The diffuseness of the mandate that they claim for themselves enables them to assert the right to set the terms on which other staff have access to patients. If the lay staff claim to have certain superior abilities, such as those made by psychologists in the area of diagnosis or by social workers in the area of family relationships, then the psychiatrist can still assert that only he can evaluate the relevance of such knowledge to the 'clinical situation'.

It may well be that there are segments and various groupings among psychiatrists, and that these make different claims for themselves. In this chapter attention has been drawn to the existence of the 'eclectics' and the 'doctors'. They may differ in the amount of importance they attach to certain activities, but both claim to possess a variety of indeterminate and technical skills. Thus routine activities such as diagnosis are imbued with a certain mystery and mystique, calling for 'intuition', 'accumulated experience' and 'clinical judgement'. By claiming to set such activities above the comprehension of non-medical staff, psychiatrists seek to maintain the subordination of the latter while at the same time striving for their compliance. It is important to stress how psychiatrists as a rule do not wish to exclude non-medical staff from contact with patients. As previously noted, some psychiatrists will readily acknowledge the ability of individual members of the non-medical staff, and will refer patients to them for therapy. However, it is also apparent that such 'recognition' is conditional upon the lay member of staff being seen to be 'reasonable', that is to have accepted those tenets of psychiatric practice that make up the medical mandate.

# 12 Sanity, Madness and the Welfare State

## by David Ingleby

Ever since the medical profession ceased to be the only one with an interest in problems of behaviour and experience, the theoretical domination of the medical model has been steadily eroded; yet it remains the fundamental paradigm of treatment within the welfare state, as if no one had ever uttered a word against it. In this chapter I shall examine the criticisms that have been made of this model, and attempt to place its use in a social and historical context. I shall argue that what we construe as mental illnesses are, if we examine them closely, manifestations of our culture and way of life; and that we seek to treat these manifestations as person-centred illnesses only because of the constraints inherent in the concept of 'welfare'.

Before going any further, however, I must briefly say what I take the medical model to be. In the *narrowest* version (sometimes also called the 'disease model'), it is assumed that the origins of the problem in question lie in some process inside the individual — an 'illness' or 'disease' — which, although it may be initiated by external or genetic causes, can be regarded as autonomous once it is in existence. In the *broadest* sense, the 'medical model' may be taken to include any approach that defines the locus of the problem as within the individual; in this sense, explanations in terms of personality or intelligence ought also to be included, especially those that claim these dispositions to be irreversible or inherited (such as Eysenck's characterlogical approach). In this chapter, I shall concentrate mainly on the disease model, though it will be obvious that much of what I shall say about this also applies to the individualistic approach in general. Moreover, although my brief is limited to so-called mental illnesses, much of what follows will also apply to physical conditions: ultimately, my criticisms are not of the illness model of psychiatry, but of the medical model of illness itself.

As I have suggested, not long ago the medical model was something on which, like the British Empire, the sun never set. Every corner of the behavioural globe was occupied by it; whatever form problems took, they could always be blamed — and usually were — on an appropriate form of 'illness'. But as far as the theoretician is concerned there is not much pink left on the map today: there are few areas of problem behaviour where the sovereignty of the medical model has not been seriously challenged.

Before examining these challenges, however, it is interesting to see how this sovereignty arose in the first place. For in the vast number of conditions which psychiatry bewilderingly calls 'functional' (as opposed to 'organic') illnesses, the criteria that justify ascribing a piece of behaviour to 'illness' in the proper sense are completely lacking; hardly ever in psychiatry is a clear pattern established of somatic causation (as opposed to somatic correlates), or of genetic (as opposed to behavioural) inheritance. Merely to establish that a particular disposition characterises an individual over time, or is associated with other characteristics, is an easier matter: but the establishment of such 'individual differences', as we shall see below, is theoretically a trivial advance.

In fact, the diagnosis of 'mental illness' is quite literally an alibi for explanation: illness is what gets invoked when a piece of behaviour cannot be understood in the normal way — it is, we might say, the default mode of explanation, now that few people believe in demons. For it is precisely when a person acts 'senselessly', 'without reason', 'incomprehensibly' or 'unintelligibly' that we start to suspect the presence of an illness. It might be thought that in saying this I am saying something completely circular — that when behaviour cannot be understood in normal terms it must be understood in abnormal terms: but what we are contrasting here, as was pointed out by Ryle (1948), are two different and mutually incompatible *modes* of understanding, rather than two kinds of factors. Roughly speaking — because this analysis is only a first approximation — our normal way of understanding behaviour is in terms of its goals or meanings (cf. the concept of 'verstehen'): the medical model, by contrast, deals only in causes. It is for this reason, therefore, that those who have set out to show the medical model's story about the causes of behaviour to be irrelevant have usually done so by claiming that the behaviour in question could be accounted for in terms of goals and meanings after all, so that a causal explanation was not necessary. (Clearly, in order to do this it will be necessary to extend our awareness of the reasons people can have for doing things: for had we regarded the behaviour as understandable in the first place, we would never have sought an illness to explain it.)

This, then, suggests the first form that challenges to the medical model may take: attempts to show that the apparently disordered 'symptoms' are in fact part of a pattern of actions following the same sort of logic as avowedly normal behaviour. I shall call this approach 'redefinition of the symptoms', in contrast to 'redefinition of the causes', in which the clinical description of the behaviour is left intact, and only its causes are viewed differently.

## REDEFINITION OF THE SYMPTOMS

Restoring the intelligibility of behaviour is a harder task than it seems, since the logic of normal behaviour is something we take very much for granted: our grasp of it is tacit, rather than explicit — informal, rather than formal. Thus, the person who sets out to show that apparently 'sick' behaviour makes sense after all has an additional gap to bridge, since he has to perform by deduction what is normally done by intuition. However, this situation is changing. Harré and Secord (1972) contrast the positivistic 'old paradigm', in which behaviour is explained as the product of internal processes and forces, with the anthropomorphic 'new paradigm', in which rules, roles, goals and meanings are paramount. Goffman (1972b) describes the changed focus of interest with characteristic piquancy — 'Not, then, men and their moments. Rather moments and their men.' There are similarities here with the distinction I set out (Ingleby, 1970) between explanations in terms of 'process' and 'praxis': in these terms, 'redefinition of the symptoms' is an attempt undo the *reification* that occurs when praxis is reduced, in the medical model, to process.

The attempts that have been made to demonstrate the intelligibility of allegedly disease-produced behaviour seem to fall into two main categories, which I shall call the 'strong' and 'weak' versions. In the *strong sense*, 'redefining the symptoms' involves claiming that the key to the problem behaviour lies entirely in the objective situation of the agent. The implication is that anybody might behave in the manner observed, if they were in the same situation: that one would not have to be an unusual kind of person to react in that way. This, of course, involves making a highly complex type of intuitive judgement — there is no way in which it can be *proved* that the response observed is or is not 'normal'. However, highly persuasive *suggestions* can be made along these lines, given a suitably vivid description of the surroundings. It is the surrounding — the context — of behaviour that traditional psychiatry has so often neglected to take into account (acting on the *a priori* conviction that the problem was caused by an illness, and therefore unrelated to its context): thus, when the context is restored, it is possible that many apparently unaccountable aspects of behaviour will suddenly make sense.

This approach, which has been called by Brown (1967) the 'normalising' approach to mental disorders, appears in perhaps its purest and most persuasive form in the accounts of schizophrenic patients and their families given by Laing and Esterson (1964). In these 'phenomenological' accounts — by which the authors meant that they had not set out to describe from the point of view of any particular theoretical preconceptions — it transpired that many of the 'symptoms' displayed by the schizophrenic were either perfectly normal activities (wearing makeup, reading the Bible) which the parents' exceedingly narrow mentality could not encompass, or natural responses to the treatment meted out by parents and doctors. One aspect of the psychological environment to which the patient was seen as giving a perfectly normal response was its ambiguous, contradictory nature: 'untenable situations' were created in which the patient was subjected to a 'double-bind' — a self-contradictory demand — to which any response would be unacceptable. (I am distinguishing this from theories such as those of Lidz, 1964, or Mischler and Waxler, 1965, which regard this peculiar environment as causally responsible for a peculiar kind of mentality.) Because of the difficulty of rendering the features of what I have called the 'psychological environment' reliably measurable, there has not been much subsequent work that might confirm or refute the impression that Laing and Esterson give. However (on the one hand) Wynne *et al.* (1958) certainly found peculiarities in the type of communications characterising families of 'schizophrenic' patients as opposed to 'neurotic' ones, or normals; against this (on the other hand) Busfield (1974) has pointed out that the conflict of roles (dependent/autonomous) supposed to be at the root of these 'double-binds' is inherent in the contemporary family, which is obliged to maintain an internal ethic of collectivity but at the same time to pass on the traditional capitalist ideology of individualism and independence. What Laing and Esterson describe, according to Busfield, is not an unusual type of conflict, but an unusual breakdown of the strategies by which 'normal' families reconcile the conflicting demands.

More generally, Laing's and Esterson's work (see also Laing, 1960, 1963; Esterson, 1972) was part of a movement that set out to demonstrate that the social environment of a person who had been labelled mentally ill differed from that of other people in ways that could account for many of his observed peculiarities. The behaviour of a person is usually related to the behaviour of those around him: to this extent, 'the standard psychiatric patient is a function of the standard psychiatrist, and of the standard mental hospital' (Laing, 1960, p. 28).

The ideas of several schools of thought converge on this notion. On the one hand, psychoanalytic family therapy, of both the British school exemplified by Laing and the French school represented by Mannoni (1969), has introduced the idea that a sick family member may function as a scapegoat for the other members, enabling them to 'project' their own disturbances on to him and have them 'carried' for them: thus, families may either make a person sick (drive him crazy), or present obstacles to his recovery if something else does so. In such situations, 'being ill' may carry symbolically the more general meaning of 'ill feelings' or 'badness' itself; Siirala (1969, 1972, 1975) has described the transfer of collective burdens that occurs in both schizophrenia and depression.

Again, American sociologists studying institutions showed how the social pressures inside insane asylums laid down not only that an inmate must be sick, but also what form his sickness should take. Goffman (1972b) states: 'If you rob people of all customary means of expressing anger and alienation and put them in a place where they have never had better reason for these feelings, then the natural recourse will be to seize on what remains — situational improprieties'; his book *Asylums* (1968) remains a pioneering classic in this area. Rosenhan (1973) reported a remarkable experiment in which a group of normal volunteers infiltrated a mental hospital and experienced these pressures at first hand. Scheff (1966) developed this theme in a wider social context, in conjunction with the ideas of

Balint (1957) and others on 'normal cases', to produce the idea of mental illness as a social role; he argued that the symptoms supposed to characterise mental patients are in fact extremely widespread in the normal population (cf. Passamanick, 1961), and that these symptoms may be used simply as pretexts for assigning someone to a 'mad' role. This role, Scheff believes, is an extremely well learned stereotype, and once one is assigned to it is very hard to shake off; both conventional responses and formal recertification procedures are heavily biased towards the conclusion that the person labelled mad must *be* mad. The social response tends to encourage the performance of the role ('deviance amplification'), which leads to behaviour far more rigid and abnormal than the symptoms that provoked the original labelling. The concept of mental illness as a 'career' conveys the way in which these approaches regard it as something laid down socially in advance.

Laing's work, and the normalising approach in general, also emphasised that many psychiatric applications of the illness model were in fact nothing more than a kind of cultural policing activity, the only grounds for singling out the behaviour in question being moral disapproval of it. Szasz (1960) — who coined the phrase 'The myth of mental illness' — was perhaps the most extreme representative of this view. Another instance of it is the recent campaign, carried on at the highest levels of the Western psychiatric establishment, against the practice among Soviet psychiatrists of treating political dissidents as mentally ill. (Needless to say, the same individuals do not protest against psychiatric repression of political dissidence carried out nearer to home, for example the practice of diagnosing the rebellious behaviour of poor Negro schoolchildren as 'hyperkinesis' and treating it by chemical sedation.)

In the *weak sense*, 'redefining the symptoms' presupposes that the 'sick' person has a different viewpoint. It is not claimed that the behaviour in question is intelligible merely if we take into account the situation in which it occurs; in addition, it is necessary to suppose that the individual has a different framework of motives, beliefs and rules of conduct. This framework may be regarded as a *social* variable — something learned from the group to which the individual belongs — or a *psychological* one, arising separately in the person: the latter theory, of course, comes very close to being an elaborated kind of 'illness model'.

The *social* theorists of this persuasion (see Taylor *et al.*, 1973) usually attempt to show that the deviant behaviour is in fact perfectly normal and reasonable by the standards of the sub-culture to which the individual in question belongs: only the social distance between him and those who call him 'deviant' accounts for the latter's response. The kind of person whose cultural background is invoked by these theorists to account for his behaviour is usually a drug addict, prostitute, petty criminal or teenage delinquent. Goffman's studies of mental patients also overlap with this category, since one of the extenuating features of the environment provided by the mental hospital is the culture of staff and patients; and so does the 'family pathology' school of Lidz (1964) and others, according to which schizophrenics are merely reproducing the bizarre linguistic and emotional culture of their families.

In all these cases, the sociologist (or psychologist) has ventured into culturally alien territory and brought back information about its norms which (he claims) would alter the views of his colleagues in the medical and penal professions, if only they would take it into account. I shall argue below, however, that the researcher need not leave 'straight' society to do this kind of job; that in certain important ways its members are so out of touch with their own culture that they fail to see how many instances of 'mental illness' are in fact manifestations of that culture.

But before taking this step it is necessary to move beyond the inherent limitations of the type of accounts of 'mental illness' we have been dealing with. Typically, these accounts can only cover behaviour that a person's own fellow-men — or the person himself — is able to make sense of in their own terms. According to this paradigm — a method carried to its logical extreme by the ethnomethodologists (see Garfinkel, 1967) — the only kind of meanings or reasons that can properly be ascribed to behaviour are those that the agent is in the habit of using: when such accounts run out, the behaviour ceases to be regarded as intelligible and is handed over to the clinician for a causal explanation. Harré and Secord (1972) likewise incorporate the shortcomings as well as the advantages of 'common sense', since they accept the mentalistic myth that all behaviour is mediated consciously and through language (Ingleby, 1973). In the psychoanalytic tradition founded by Freud, however, the beliefs and goals according to which 'pathological' behaviour is alleged to make sense are ones whose existence is largely ignored or denied — a kind of unavowed sub-culture. The same search for unavowed significance was pursued, in different directions, by Marx and Nietsche — whom, with Freud, Paul Ricoeur has called one of the three 'masters of suspicion' of our age; and this phrase sums up neatly the underlying attitude to commonsense interpretations of behaviour.

Psychoanalysis, then, offers an 'interpretation' of apparently mysterious, bizarre or preposterous behaviour in terms of what is, in a sense, a kind of sub-culture — a system of unacknowledged wishes, beliefs and scenarios (Laing's term) known as 'primary process' or 'unconscious phantasy'. Even behaviour that appears quite straightforward on the surface can be given, according to psychoanalysis, an alternative interpretation in these terms. Unlike the sub-cultures unearthed by the sociologists of deviance, however, whose relevance was not appreciated because they were distant and unknown, the unconscious system is not invoked (the psychoanalysts say) because it is too close for comfort: precisely because unconscious phantasy operates in everybody is there a 'resistance' to acknowledging its operations.

Psychoanalysis identifies the world of the mentally ill with the magical world of the child: the beliefs and wishes that have to be imputed to make sense of disturbed behaviour are not (as many suppose) inferred purely *ad hoc*, but form a coherent system which can be observed both in its original and its archaeological forms, in the child and the adult. It was, in fact, Melanie Klein (1948) who made the most detailed study of the prototypes of 'pathological' thought in the very young child. The extent to which a person acts in accordance with the unconscious system is taken as the index of his 'mental health'; such disturbances as neuroses or psychoses merely represent varying degrees of 'regression to' or 'fixation at' this stage of thinking.

We see thus that psychoanalysis is an extension of commonsense ways of explaining behaviour, in so far as it invokes meanings and purposes rather than causes; however, the analyst restores meaning to disturbed behaviour only at a price — the price of acknowledging that the behaviour makes sense only in the context of a world that is not the one we like to think of as normal, adult reality. Thus, psychoanalysis fills out Wittgenstein's saying (1972, p. 147) that 'the world of the happy man is a different one from that of the unhappy man'. What remains to be explained, however, after the interpretations have been made, is *why* a person comes to find himself in this world; and it is to fulfil this function that the concept of mental illness is usually invoked. The illness may be regarded as 'caused' by immediate or long-buried events, or simply by constitutional factors.

We seem here to have arrived back at a view in which 'person-variables' are supreme: psychoanalysis emphasises the extent to which past experience conditions present experience, so that a person with unresolved problems at the level of unconscious phantasy will not thrive even in a benign environment, and a person free of such problems will cope even in the hardest conditions. Such a theory could easily be used, like the Victorian religious approach to life, as a reason for doing nothing to ameliorate people's environments; and in the training of social workers it is often used to this effect. It is Mr Smith's oedipal problems, rather than unemployment or bad housing, that are held responsible for the plight of his 'multi-problem' family: the *real* problems are 'all in the mind'. Yet it seems to me that this interpretation of the psychoanalytic model, however widely accepted in England and America, does not accord even with the view of its originator, Freud, who regarded psychoanalysis as a subversive, almost 'criminal', activity.

For psychoanalysis can be reduced to a simple illness model, with all the reactionary consequences this entails, only if certain facts of life are ignored. The crucial issue concerns the origin of the beliefs and goals that constitute unconscious phantasy. The illness model seeks to show that these are created simply as defence mechanisms to protect the individual from certain painful realities; for example, a man may harbour the wish to become an inseparable part of another person, along with phantasies of getting 'right inside', which are regularly acted out in sexual intercourse, as a defence against the pain of being separate. While this may be true in the first instance, it is also true that these defence mechanisms may be powerfully reinforced by both the family environment and the wider culture. Thus, the notion that mental illness represents a switch from adult reality to primitive infantile thinking is based on a false distinction; for 'adult reality', when closely examined, turns out to contain many of the magical and mythical elements supposed to characterise childhood.

In the family context, such therapists as Mannoni (1969), Laing (1960) and Lidz (1964) have emphasised — as we saw above — that the patients' 'delusions' may constitute part of the family mythology;

thus, a patient might have phantasies of being a part of his mother, so that she can feel his pain, know his mind and know what he 'really' wants — and these phantasies might very well turn out to be accepted beliefs within the family. At the cultural level less systematic work has been undertaken, but I would argue that there is sufficient evidence to reject the view that the neurotic or psychotic mentality is solely a product of individual or family pathology. It is not simply that (*pace* Scheff and Passamanick) symptoms of psychopathology are extremely prevalent in the normal population: the very notion that 'normal' behaviour is 'rational' is itself one of the guiding myths of psychiatry. Practically every feature of the thinking that analysts isolate in their 'sick' patients has its counterpart in some social institution or belief.

Certain delusions and illusory goals are, in fact, actively fostered to provide the motive force of social organisation. Oedipal strivings motivate a man's career ambition; oral cravings make him a willing and easily led consumer; separation anxiety makes him eager to attach himself to a firm, a family or a cause. For most people who work, 'the job' becomes delusionally equated with their own anti-libidinal tendencies; only thus can its demands acquire the inexorable and inhuman authority that they have for the average person, making work one of the 'institutionalised forms of suicide' of which Sirola (1975) writes. What has been called the 'normal psychosis' of being in love furnishes the pretext, if not the mainstay, of most marriages; while splitting and projection maintain the division of labour and the roles of leaders, criminals, foreigners and women. Pre-psychotic phantasies of persecution by dirt send the housewife scurrying to the supermarket for detergents that can never remove the stain — because the stain is 'in the mind': any competent marketing executive could no doubt fill a book with further examples. Thus, such 'defences' are (as Freud would have put it) 'overdetermined', in that they have a function in the two intersecting domains of psychic and social economy: they both act as emotional defences for the individual, and facilitate his social exploitation. The treadmill of compulsions that most of us turn daily may be constructed out of our own private fears and woes, but it is carefully oiled and harnessed by the maintenance men of modern industrial civilisation.

Many of the problems that the psychoanalytic patient needs helping with, therefore, are problems that he has by virtue of being a member of this culture. For instance, one of the tasks of analysis is to learn to treat oneself and others as people — that is dialectically, rather than in the depersonalised, reified way of the child to whom the mother is just an object to be sucked. The ultimate irony, as Siirala (1969) has pointed out, is that clinical medicine itself — to which the 'dehumanised' psychiatric patient comes to be cured — is itself the ultimately reified and depersonalised mentality. Thus, the goals of the psychoanalyst are bound to come into conflict with social organisation at this point — for to make out in society as it is, it is *necessary* to treat oneself and others as objects rather than as people. Furthermore, part of the process of becoming a person is accepting responsibility for one's own life; but in many areas — especially the political — people socially are required to think of themselves as perpetual children.

Therefore, to speculate about the causes of regression and fixation without considering the way in which the individual's culture colludes with these defences — in other words, to treat psychoanalysis as a purely psychological or medical specialty — is shortsighted. As long as dreams and nightmares furnish so much of the logic of our daily social transactions, we cannot regard Freudian psychopathology as the hallmark of deviance or illness. As it happens, Freud seems to have been aware of all this; and the present-day requirement that all analysts should themselves have been patients is a very curious one unless we are to infer that every analyst, by virtue of being a normal citizen, has something to be cured of.

With this insight, the explanatory power of psychoanalysis diminishes sharply — for if 'unconscious phantasy' is ubiquitous, it cannot explain what is specifically wrong with the mental patient; but at the same time, its potential as a social critique increases. Clearly, the liberation of the patient from his illusions involves undoing much of his socialisation, if these illusions are collective ones: it is in this sense that I believe Freud thought of psychoanalysis as a 'criminal' kind of activity. Moreover, this task of liberation must be a political as well as a psychological one: the 'resistances' encountered will be of a double nature, for as well as the Freudian ones there will also be the kind that Goldmann wrote about: 'For there are also elements of reality essential to the existence of a class which it is not in the interests of that class to have subjected to public, or even scientific, scrutiny. Anyone seeking to study such elements will encounter powerful internal and external resistances' (1969, p. 43).

It was not only Freud, but Marx as well, who described the ways in which the real nature of transactions between people is masked by the distorted representations — ideologies — through which man represents to himself his own activities. (Where neuroses and ideologies most actively collude, perhaps, is in misrepresenting the nature of, and denying the importance of, our transactions with each other: in masking human needs and human pain.) Therefore, in so far as certain illusions serve a double (personal and political) function, the task of the psychoanalyst is the *same* as that of the analyst of ideology; not merely, as I suggested in an earlier paper (Ingleby, 1974a), *similar* to it.

REDEFINITION OF THE CAUSES

At first sight it would not appear to constitute a major attack on the medical model if one accepts the reality of the symptoms, as medically defined, but merely ascribes them to something other than internal pathology. This revised etiology, however, does make a radical difference, for the simple reason that 'illness' is more than a purely descriptive category: it not only defines one's condition, but hypothesises an internal process responsible for it. (For instance, it would be obviously unfair to describe the emaciation of concentration camp prisoners as 'illness' — although they are undeniably not 'well'.) Confusion arises because we lack a sharper distinction between the observable facts of 'dis-ease' and 'ill-ness' and the factors responsible for them — which may or may not be autonomous internal processes: in other words, a purely descriptive criterion of wellbeing.

In the light of their causes, many conditions traditionally regarded as mental illnesses turn out to be perhaps not illnesses at all — despite the fact that they may be associated with as much suffering and disturbance of functioning as the concentration camp conditions mentioned above. For example, the widespread incidence of depression among housewives or production-line workers may simply be due to the fact that their lives are, in fact, depressing; similarly, the executive suffering from symptoms of insecurity may in reality be living a very insecure existence. The same type of argument may be applied to the equally relentless phenomena of senile depressions, psychoses and confusional states; as Kastenbaum (1970) has pointed out, it is a reasonable hypothesis that, leaving aside any organic process of 'ageing', any person would be confused, depressed and maddened by the experiences that an ageing person must endure. It would be more accurate to say that reality retreats from the elderly than that they retreat from it.

At this point it would be nice to be able to adduce plentiful empirical evidence to show the importance of 'environmental factors' in mental illness. The data we need, however, are missing; and I believe they are missing not because there are no such factors, but because our standard methodology is biased in two important ways against them and in favour of individual factors.

First, it is no great discovery that individual differences exist in people's vulnerability to pathogenic environmental conditions: few biological phenomena occur in an all-or-none manner. Thus, there always will exist person-variables as well as situation-variables in the determination of 'illness'. But the decision as to which of these are regarded as the 'cause' will not reflect their relative potency, but the purely pragmatic question of which variable one prefers to manipulate: in other words, a 'variable' comes to mean 'that which may be varied' (Ingleby, 1974b). This choice will depend on the context. Let us take as an example the joint contribution of body temperature and anoxia to human tissue survival. If we are talking about a death by strangulation, we will obviously consider anoxia to be the cause of death, rather than the fact that the victim's body temperature was normal — although he might have survived at a lower temperature: in that situation, body temperature was not easily varied, so it is not regarded as a cause. If, however, we are talking about a surgical operation in which breathing is halted, performed under hypothermia, we would equally obviously say that a rise in body temperature was responsible for death, if the apparatus regulating it failed: here, the anoxia would not be the 'cause', because it was not the easiest factor to vary. As I shall show later, the traditional emphasis in medicine on manipulating person-variables rather than situation-variables leads to the habit of regarding only the former as 'causes': in other words, we regard the person as the 'cause' of the problem only because it is the person we prefer to treat rather than his environment.

Second, even when the selection of 'causes' is based on research rather than treatment priorities, the bias is still away from environmental factors and in favour of the illness model. Typically, the researcher estimates the relative contribution to a condition of different factors by comparing the variance that each of them accounts for (as, for instance, in estimates of the 'heritability' of intelligence quotients). However, the amount of variance that a given factor accounts for will depend not only on the influence that it exerts on the dependent variable, but on the degree to which it varies in the sample under consideration — a parameter that is usually left unquantified. Such investigations will tend to mask the effect of the factors that all the members of a sample have in common, such as — at the most general level — their way of life as a function of their geographical location and historical epoch. If everybody were on a bad diet, for example, then the variance in metabolic disorders could be accounted for only by individual differences, and nobody might ever realise what was wrong. Similarly, the inadequacies of the environmental 'diet' provided by modern industrial civilisation as a whole might never come to light if only visible variations were studied. And it is not only psychiatric medicine that is biased against the recognition of collective social causes: for exactly the same pragmatic and statistical reasons, physical medicine shows this complicity with current social conditions. When a doctor certifies that the death of a patient was due to 'natural causes', he is including in the concept of 'nature' a whole host of conditions — housing, labour, interpersonal relationships — which are not really part of 'nature' at all, but part of the man-made artefact called 'civilisation'.

What the study of environmental factors requires, then, is a form of analysis that will place 'illness' firmly in its historical context. Foucault (1967) attempted to do this, for the incidence of madness in the classical age: his analysis has been penetratingly applied by the literary critic Tony Tanner (1969) to Jane Austen's *Sense and Sensibility* — a novel that describes both a typical form of eighteenth-century 'nervous disorder' and the social conditions which gave rise to it. For the present age, however, few writers of any substance have attempted an analysis comparable to Foucault's. The only studies I know of that have attempted to relate psychiatric conditions to their historical context in any detail are Fanon's (1970) study of colonial life, and Maucorps' (1970) essay on the 'social vacuum', which drives many rural inhabitants in the surroundings of Paris temporarily insane. Siirala's work, cited above, is also a noteworthy step in the same direction.

## THE ROLE OF WELFARE

To appreciate how the social role of medicine makes it impossible to escape, in practice, from the limitations of the medical model, we have only to consider how our attitude to psychiatric problems would be altered by the adoption of the different perspectives I have been examining.

Firstly, we note that a change is implied in the status of the person who was previously regarded as harbouring the problem. An element of submission is always associated with the treatment of pathological conditions: in the first place there can be no arguing about the desirability of having the condition removed (hence the extraordinary moral force of the 'illness' label), and in the second place the 'sick' person, by definition, lacks the physical and mental capacity to look after himself properly. There can therefore be no question of equality in decision-making between the patient and the medical agency. In contrast, when the medical model is abandoned, quite different attitudes to the 'patient' become appropriate — depending on the alternative model adopted.

When we 'redefine the symptoms', we are adopting an anthropomorphic model, i.e. 'treating people as people'; and the double meaning of this phrase is significant. In such a model, 'seeing the other person's point of view' becomes a formally necessary scientific operation — for it is in terms of his point of view that we attempt to understand his behaviour. In the 'normalising' approach — that is, when we attempt to show that the behaviour in question is perfectly appropriate when its context is fully appreciated — it immediately becomes important to ask why the behaviour is regarded as a problem in the first place — who it is a problem for, and why. (Consider, for example, the hospitalised members of Laing's sample of families; the 'insane' Soviet dissenters; or the 'hyperkinetic' Negro children.) In the weak sense of 'redefining the symptoms', when behaviour is claimed to be justifiable in terms of the agent's point of view, we have to establish why one point of view is to be given precedence over another. Who has the more viable framework — the slum criminal or the middle-class social worker; the 'regressed' patient or the 'well-adjusted' therapist? Lastly, when we merely redefine the cause of a condition agreed to be unhealthy in terms that place the blame on factors external to the individual, it becomes irrelevant (except for purposes of first aid) to apply treatment to the individual himself and not to his situation.

I hope by this point to have illustrated the contrast between the medical model and its alternatives clearly enough to show what a conceptual prison it has become. One would expect from this that those inside the prison would have welcomed their liberators with open arms, but these theorists have mostly been given a hostile reception. Consequently, we find the medical model at the root of every activity of the welfare, educational and penal agencies. Even where psychiatric methods have changed away from traditional medical practice — for example, in 'community care', behaviour therapy or social work — we still find the same talk of 'treatment plans' and the same emphasis on modifying the patient (or the 'client', as he is sometimes ironically described) rather than his surroundings. The latest research plans of the most prestigious institutions — the Tavistock Institute, or the Institute of Psychiatry — are concerned with identifying individual characteristics that can be held responsible for delinquency, crime, school failure and poverty. One might imagine that this is due to the inevitable time lag in the distribution of ideas, but the ideas have been distributed long ago; it is not worth waiting for the penny to drop, because the real reason for the persistence of the medical model lies in the nature of the health agencies themselves.

In other words, I am arguing that these agencies cannot adapt to the types of alternative theory that I have outlined, because the implementation of these theories would require too radical a break with their social role. Let us examine, therefore, what this social role is. In Britain today it is compounded of the traditions of private medicine and the concept of the welfare state. Now the role of private medicine has always been such as to focus treatment on the individual: what is not generally appreciated is that the employee of the welfare state — for different reasons — works under the same constraints. From the outset, the welfare services were conceived of not as autonomous agencies devoted to the general wellbeing of the population, but as back-up services for a particular form of social organisation: they have no brief for initiating, or even recommending, any change in the form of this organisation itself. The welfare worker, then, has quite literally no use for theories that imply the need for social change: he is as unlikely to develop and apply such theories as the medieval clergy would have been to develop and apply the contraceptive pill. Conversely, the theories that he does have a use for are those that concentrate on short-term, individual remedies for problems, and do not raise the questions of why they are problems in the first place, or how they are rooted in social conditions. The medical model serves in important ways to stabilise and justify the *status quo*: it is ideally suited to the removal of the disturbing problems that arise at the tension points of the modern state. Clearly, as Sedgewick (1973) has argued, it is neither humane nor revolutionary to leave the casualties of the State unattended on the street: but it is equally true, as the Women's Movement has effectively insisted, that the use of tranquillisers and ECT to enforce acceptance of intolerable conditions is downright oppressive.

Again, by implying that the real inadequacies lie in the 'problem' individuals, the medical model condones the inadequate conditions in which their deficiencies become manifest. Joanna Ryan (in Chapter 10) has pointed out how the categorisation of children as 'mentally subnormal' seems to be determined by the requirements of the labour market; and the policy of removing such children from their families and placing them in institutions is determined by the economic and cultural limitations placed on what families can and cannot do. The medical model, however, has effectively disguised these realities by inventing a clinical category of 'subnormality' and making hospitalisation a *medical* imperative. But nowhere is this strategy more apparent than in the current debate about the 'cycle of deprivation' — a conceptual invention on the investigation of which increasing amounts of public money are being spent. It is interesting to examine the original speech by Sir Keith Joseph (1972), then Minister of Health, as a piece of entirely orthodox ideology. (I am indebted to an unpublished paper by Sue Holland, formerly of the Tavistock Clinic, for many of these observations.) Because deprivation is due to individual factors as well as socioeconomic ones, Sir Keith argues that the persistence of deprivation 'despite all our advances' must be due to the former, i.e. to weak families or genes: he does not stop to consider the possibility that some of our 'advances' on the social front may be more imaginary than real. Of the two types of factors admitted to be relevant, only individual factors are regarded as variables (i.e. open to being varied), and hence are conceptualised as 'causes'; socioeconomic circumstances are treated as constants established by the laws of nature — a myth that is unwittingly uttered by Sir Keith when he goes on to speak of 'young children and their parents *destined* [my italics] to live in bleak urban areas'. Sir Keith speaks of 'fundamentally preventative measures of social policy', and of 'getting back to root causes', but it turns out that what he is talking about is strengthening vulnerable individuals by improving patterns of child-rearing: doing this is no more a 'radical' solution to the problems created by our system of social ·organisation than the provision of computerised fingerprint scanners and radio-controlled anti-hijacking devices is a 'radical' solution to the problem of crime.

If the gist of this paper is correct, therefore, I would argue that research and action on the social roots of the problems now dealt with by medical and paramedical agencies cannot be entrusted to the machinery of the welfare state, as it is defined at present. If medical sociology is to do anything more radical than merely study the sociology of existing medical practice — if it is to achieve a synthesis, rather than merely a sum, of sociology and medicine — it must do so within a framework that does not harbour the limitations of perspective and policy that I have outlined.

# Bibliography

Adams, J. (1973) 'Adaptive behaviour and measured intelligence in the classification of mental retardation' *Amer. J. Ment. Defic.* 78, p. 77.

Anderson, E. M. (1973) *The Disabled Schoolchild: A Study of Integration in Primary Schools* London, Methuen.

Atkinson, P., Reid, M. and Sheldrake, P. (1972) *Medical Mystique: Indeterminacy and Models of Professional Process* Occasional Paper No. 14, Centre for Research in Education and Science, University of Edinburgh.

Bales, R. F. (1951) *Interaction Process Analysis* Reading, Mass., Addison-Wesley.

Balint, M. (1957) *The Doctor, His Patient and the Illness* London, Pitman.

Barclay, A. and Vaught, G. (1964) 'Maternal estimates of future achievement in cerebral palsied children' *Amer. J. Ment. Def.* 69, p. 62.

Bayley, M. (1973) *Mental Handicap and Community Care* London, Routledge & Kegan Paul.

Becker, H. S. (1963) *Outsiders: Studies in the Sociology of Deviance* Glencoe, Ill., Free Press.

Becker, H. S. (1970) *Sociological Work* Chicago, Aldine.

Bijou, S. W. (1967) 'A functional analysis of retarded development' in N. R. Ellis (ed.) *International Review of Research in Mental Retardation* (vol. 1) New York, Academic Press.

Birch, H. O., Belmont, L., Belmont, I. and Taft, L. (1967) 'Brain damage in educable mentally subnormal children' *J. Neur. Ment. Dis.* 144, p. 247.

Birdwhistell, R. C. (1973) *Kinesics and Context: Essays on Body-Motion Communication* Harmondsworth, Penguin.

Birenbaum, A. (1970) 'On managing a courtesy stigma' *J. Health and Soc. Behav.* 11, p. 196.

Boles, G. (1959) 'Personality factors in mothers of cerebral palsied children' *Genet. Psychol. Mongr.* 59, p. 159.

*British Medical Journal* (1972) 'Febrile Convulsions in Early Childhood' (Leader, 10 June).

Brown, G. W. (1967) 'The family of the schizophrenic patient' in A. Coppen and A. Walk (eds) *Recent Developments in Schizophrenia* London, Royal Medico-Psychological Association.

Busfield, J. (1974) 'Family ideology and family pathology' in N. Armistead (ed.) *Reconstructing Social Psychology* Harmondsworth, Penguin.

Caron, H. S. and Roth, H. P. (1968) 'Patients' co-operation with a medical regimen' *J. Amer. Med. Assoc.* 203, p. 922.

Cartwright, A. (1966) *Patients and their Doctors* London, Routledge & Kegan Paul.

Cartwright, A. (1968) 'General practitioners and family planning' *Med. Offr.* 120, p. 43.

Cicourel, A. (1973) *Cognitive Sociology* Harmondsworth, Penguin.

Clarke, A. D. B. and Clarke A. M. (1973a) 'Assessment and prediction' in P. Mittler (ed.) *Assessment for Learning in the Mentally Handicapped* London, Churchill Livingstone.

Clarke, A. D. B. and Clarke, A. M. (eds) (1973b) *Mental Retardation and Behavioural Research* London, Churchill Livingstone.

212

Clarke, A. M. and Clarke, A. D. B. (eds) (1958) *Mental Deficiency, The Changing Outlook* London, Methuen.

Clausen, J. (1966) *Ability Structure and Subgroups in Mental Retardation* London, Macmillan.

Cooper, D. (1967) *Psychiatry and Anti Psychiatry* London, Tavistock Publications.

Crome, L. and Stern, J. (1967) *The Pathology of Mental Retardation* London, Churchill Livingstone.

Davis, F. (1960) 'Uncertainty in medical prognosis: clinical and functional' *Amer. J. Soc.* 66, p. 41.

Dembo, T. (1964) 'Sensitivity of one person to another' *Rehab. Lit.* 25, p. 231.

Denzin, N. K. (1971) 'Symbolic interactionism and ethnomethodology' in J. D. Douglas (ed.) *Understanding Everyday Life* London, Routledge & Kegan Paul.

DHSS (1971) *Better Services for the Mentally Handicapped* London, HMSO.

Dingwall, R. W. J. (1974) 'The social organisation of health visitor training' Unpublished PhD thesis, University of Aberdeen.

Douglas, J. D. (1967) *The Social Meaning of Suicide* Princeton, N.J., University Press.

Douglas, J. D. (ed.) (1971) *Understanding Everyday Life* London, Routledge & Kegan Paul.

Duff, R. and Hollingshead, A. B. (1968) *Sickness and Society* New York, Harper & Row.

Edgerton, R. (1965) 'Some dimensions of disillusionment in culture contact' *South Western Journal of Anthropology* 21, p. 231.

Edgerton, R. B. (1970) 'Mental retardation in non-Western societies' in H. C. Haywood (ed.) *Social-Cultural Aspects of Mental Retardation* New York, Appleton.

Ellis, N. R. (ed.) (1963) *Handbook of Mental Deficiency* New York, McGraw Hill.

Ellis, N. R. (1969) 'A behavioural research strategy in mental retardation: defense and critique' *Amer. J. Ment. Defic.* 73, p. 557.

Emerson, R. (1969) *Judging Delinquents, Context and Process in a Juvenile Court* Chicago, Aldine.

Esterson, A. (1972) *The Leaves of Spring: a Study in the Dialectics of Madness* London, Tavistock Publications.

Fanon, F. (1970) *Black Skin, White Masks* London, Paladin.

Farber, B. (1968) *Mental Retardation: its Social Context and Social Consequences* Boston, Houghton Mifflin.

Festinger, L. (1957) *A Theory of Cognitive Dissonance* New York, Row, Peterson.

Filmer, P., Philipson, M., Silverman, D. and Walsh, D. *New Directions in Sociological Theory* London, Collier Macmillan.

Firth, J. R. (1957) 'The techniques of semantics' (1935) in *Papers in Linguistics 1934-51* London, Oxford University Press.

Fletcher, C. (1974) *Beneath the Surface: an Account of Three Styles of Sociological Research* London, Routledge & Kegan Paul.

Flexner, A. (1915) 'Is social work a profession?' in *Proceedings of the National Conference of Charities and Correction* Chicago, Hildmann Printing.

Ford, A. B., Liske, R. E., Ort, R. S. and Dewton, J. C. (1967) *The Doctor's Perspective* Cleveland, Case Western Reserve University.

Foucault, M. (1967) *Madness and Civilisation* London, Tavistock Publications.

Freidson, E. (1970) *Professional Dominance: The Social Structure of Medical Care* New York, Atherton Press.

Freidson, E. (1971) *The Profession of Medicine* New York, Dodd and Mead.

Garfinkel, H. (1964) 'Studies of the routine grounds of everyday activities' *Social Problems* 11, p. 3.

Garfinkel, H. (1967) *Studies in Ethnomethodology* Englewood Cliffs, N.J., Prentice-Hall.

Gill, D. G. and Horobin, G. W. (1972) 'Doctors, patients and the State: relationships and decision-making' *Soc. Rev.* 20, p. 505.

Goffman, E. (1961) *Encounters* New York, Bobbs-Merrill.

Goffman, E. (1963) *Stigma* Englewood Cliffs, N.J., Prentice Hall.

Goffman, E. (1968) *Asylums* Harmondsworth, Penguin.

Goffman, E. (1971) *The Presentation of Self in Everyday Life* Harmondsworth, Penguin.

Goffman, E. (1972a) *Interaction Rituals* Harmondsworth, Penguin.

Goffman, E. (1972b) *Relations in Public* Harmondsworth, Penguin.

Goldberg, D. (1972) 'Psychiatry and general practice' *Medicine* 9, p. 630.

Goldie, N. (1974) 'Professional Processes Among Three Occupational Groups Within the Mental Health Field' Unpublished PhD thesis, The City University, London.

Goldmann, L. (1969) *Philosophy and the Human Sciences* London, Cape.

Gunzberg, H. C. (1973) 'The role of the psychologist in "manipulating" the institutional environment' in A. D. B. Clarke and A. M. Clarke (eds.) *Mental Retardation and Behavioural Research* London, Churchill Livingstone.

Harré R. and Secord, P. F. (1972) *The Explanation of Social Behaviour* Oxford, Blackwell.

Henry, W. E., Sims, J. and Spray, S. (1971) *The Fifth Profession — Becoming a Psychotherapist* San Francisco, Jossey-Bass.

HMSO (1969) *People with Epilepsy* (The Reid Report) London, Her Majesty's Stationery Office.

Hebb, D. O. (1949) *The Organisation of Behaviour* New York, Wiley.

Hewett, S. (1970) *The Family and the Handicapped Child* London, Allen and Unwin.

Hill, D. (1969) *Psychiatry in Medicine* London, Oxford University Press for Nuffield Provincial Hospital Trust.

Holt, K. S. and Huntley, R. M. C. (1973) 'Mental subnormality: medical training in the United Kingdom' *Brit. J. Med. Educ.* 7, p. 197.

Horobin, G. and Bloor, M. J. (1975) 'Role-taking in illness' in Caroline Cox and Adrienne Mead (eds) *The Sociology of Medical Practice* London, Macmillan.

Hsia, D. (1967) 'Y-Y. The hereditary metabolic diseases' in J. Hirsch (ed.) *Behaviour-Genetic Analysis* New York, McGraw Hill.

Illich, I. (1973) 'The professions as a form of imperialism' *New Society* (13 September).

Ima, K., Tagliacozzo, D. M. and Lashof, J. C. (1970) 'Physician orientation and behaviour' *Med. care* 8, p. 189.

Ingleby, J. D. (1970) 'Ideology and the human sciences' *The Human Context* 2, p. 159.

Ingleby, J. D. (1973) 'New paradigms for old' *Radical Philosophy* 6, p. 42.

Ingleby, J. D. (1974a) 'The psychology of child psychology' in M. Richards (ed.) *The Integration of a Child into a Social World* Cambridge, University Press.

Ingleby, J. D. (1974b) 'The job psychologists do' in N. Armistead (ed.) *Reconstructing Social Psychology* Harmondsworth, Penguin.

Jamous, H. and Peliolle, B. (1970) 'Professions or self perpetuating systems. Changes in the French University Hospital Service' in J. Jackson (ed.) *Professions and Professionalisation* Cambridge, University Press.

Jensen, A. R. (1970) 'A theory of primary and secondary familial mental retardation' in N. R. Ellis (ed.) *International Review of Research in Mental Retardation* (vol. 4) New York, Academic Press.

Jensen, G. D. and Kogan, K. L. (1962) 'Parental estimates of the future achievement of children with cerebral palsy' *J. Ment. Def. Res.* 6, p. 56.

Joseph, K. (1972) speech delivered on 29 June 1972 at a conference of local authorities organised by the Pre-School Playgroups Association.

Joyce, C. R. B., Caple, G., Mason, M., Reynolds, E. and Mathews, J. A. (1969) 'Quantitative study of doctor—patient communication' *Quart. J. Med.* 38, p. 183.

Kanner, L. (1964) *A History of the Care and Study of the Mentally Retarded* Springfield, Ill., C. C. Thomas.

Kastenbaum, R. (1970) 'Theoretical models and model theoreticians in gerontology' in D. P. Kent, R. Kastenbaum and S. Sherwood (eds.) *Research, Planning and Action for the Elderly* New York, Behavioural Publications.

Keith, R. A. and Markie, G. S. (1969) 'Parental and professional assessment of functioning in cerebral palsy' *Devel. Med. and Child Neurol.* 11, p. 735.

Kennedy, D. A., (1973) 'Perceptions of illness and healing' *Soc. Sci. and Med.* 7, p. 787.

King, R. D., Raynes, N. V. and Tizard, J. (1971) *Patterns of Residential Care* London, Routledge & Kegan Paul.

Klein, M. (1948) *Contributions to Psycho-analysis, 1921-45* London, Hogarth Press.

Korsch, B. and Negrete, V. F. (1972) 'Doctor—patient communication' *Scientific American* 227, p. 66.

Laing, R. D. (1960) *The Divided Self* London, Tavistock Publications.

Laing, R. D. (1963) *The Self and Others* London, Tavistock Publications.

Laing, R. D. and Esterson, A. (1964) *Families of Schizophrenics* London, Tavistock Publications.

Leck, I., Gordon, W. L. and McKeown, T. (1967) 'Medical and social needs of patients in hospitals for the mentally subnormal' *Brit. J. Prev. Soc. Med.* 21, p. 115.

Lemert, E. (1968) 'Paranoia and the dynamics of exclusion' in E. Rubington and M. S. Weinberg (eds) *Deviance, the Interactionist Perspective* London, Macmillan.

Ley, P. (1972) 'Primacy, rated importance and the recall of medical statements' *J. Hlth. & Soc. Behav.* 13, p. 311.

Ley, P. and Spelman, M. S. (1965) 'Communications in an out-patient setting' *Brit. J. Soc. Clinc. Psych.* 4, p. 114.

Lidz, T. (1964) *The Family and Human Adaptation* London, Hogarth Press.

Manning, P. K. (1972) in J. D. Douglas (ed.) *Research on Deviance* New York, Random House.

Mannoni, M. (1969) *The Child, his Illness, and the Family* London, Tavistock Publications.

Martin, H. W. (1962) 'Structural sources of strain in a small psychiatric hospital' *Psychiatry* 25, p. 4.

Marx, J. H. (1969) 'A multidimensional conception of ideology in the professional arena' *Pacific Sociological Review* 3, p. 101.

Maucorps, P. (1970) 'Social vacuum' *The Human Context* 2, p. 31.

Mauksch, H. O. (1972) 'Ideology, interaction and patient care in hospitals' paper presented at the Third International Conference on Social Science and Medicine, Elsinore, Denmark.

McQueen, I. A. G. (1962) 'From carbolic powder to social counsel' (centenary address to Battersea College of Technology) *Nursing Times* 58, p. 866.

Mead, G. H. (1934) *Mind, Self and Society* Chicago, University Press.

Mercer, J. R. (1973) *Labelling the Mentally Retarded* Berkeley, University of California Press.

Meyersohn, R. (1969) *Sociology and Cultural Studies: Some Problems.* Occasional Paper No. 5, Centre for Contemporary Cultural Studies, Birmingham University.

Millichap, J. G. (1968) *Febrile Convulsions* New York, Macmillan.

Mischler, E. G. and Waxler, N. E. (1965) 'Family interaction processes and schizophrenia: a review of current theories' *Merrill-Palmer Quarterly* 2, p. 269.

Mittler, P. (1973) 'Purposes and principles of assessment' in P. Mittler (ed.) *Assessment for Learning in the Mentally Handicapped* London, Churchill Livingstone.

Moerman, M. (1974) 'Accomplishing ethnicity' in R. Turner (ed.) *Ethnomethodology* Harmondsworth, Penguin.

O'Connor, N. and Hermelin, B. (1963) *Speech and Thought in Severe Subnormality* London, Pergamon.

Opie, I. and Opie, P. (1967) *The Lore and Language of Schoolchildren* Oxford, University Press.

Opie, I. and Opie, P. (1970) *Games Children Play* Oxford, University Press.

Parsons, T. (1951) *The Social System* New York, Free Press.

Parsons, T. (1954) *Essays in Sociological Theory* Glencoe, Ill., Free Press.

Parsons, T. (1964) *Social Structure and Personality* Glencoe, Ill., Free Press.

Passamanick, B. (1961) 'A survey of mental disease in an urban population: IV. An approach to total prevalence rates' *Archives of General Psychiatry* 5, p. 151.

Penrose, L. S. (1963) *The Biology of Mental Defect* (3rd ed.) London, Sidgwick.

Penrose, L. S. and Smith, G. F. (1966) *Down's Anomaly* London, Churchill Livingstone.

Pilling, D. (1972) *The Orthopaedically Handicapped Child. Social, Emotional and Educational Adjustment: An Annotated Bibliography* Windsor, Berks., NFER.

Pilling, D. (1973a) *The Child with Cerebral Palsy. Social, Emotional and Educational Adjustment: An Annotated Bibliography* Windsor, Berks., NFER.

Pilling, D. (1973b) *The Child with Spina Bifida. Social, Emotional and Educational Adjustment: An Annotated Bibliography* Windsor, Berks., NFER.

Pratt, L., Seligmann, A. and Reader, G. (1957) 'Physicians' views on the level of medical information among patients' *Am. J. publ. Hlth.* 47, p. 1277.

Pringle, M. L. K. and Fiddes, D. O. (1970) *The Challenge of Thalidomide* London, Longman.

Pritchard, D. G. (1963) *Education and the Handicapped 1760-1960* London, Routledge & Kegan Paul.

Richards, B. W. (ed.) (1970) *Mental Subnormality: Modern Trends in Research* London, Pitman.

Robinson, D. (1971) *The Process of Becoming Ill* London, Routledge & Kegan Paul.

Robinson, D. (1976) *From Drinking to Alcoholism: a Sociological Commentary* London, John Wiley.

Robinson, H. B. and Robinson N. M. (1965) *The Mentally Retarded Child* New York, McGraw Hill.

Rosen, H. (1972) *Language and Class: a Critical Look at the Theories of Basil Bernstein* Bristol, Falling Wall Press.

Rosenhan, D. L. (1973) 'On being sane in insane places' *Science* 179, p. 250.

Roskies, E. (1972) *Abnormality and Normality: The Mothering of Thalidomide Children* Ithaca, N. Y., Cornell University Press.

Ross, E. M. (1974) 'A Bristol study of secondary school children' unpublished MD thesis, Bristol University Medical School.

Roth, J. (1971) 'Utilization of the hospital emergency department' *J. Health Soc. Beh.* 12, p. 312.

Roth, J. A. (1974) 'Professionalism: the sociologists decoy' *Sociology of Work and Occupations* 1, p. 6.

Royal College of General Practitioners (1972) *The Future General Practitioner* London, RCGP.

Ryan, J. F. (1971) 'Classification and behaviour in mental subnormality' in D. Primrose (ed.) *Proceedings of 1st Congress of International Association for Study of Mental Deficiency* Warsaw, Polish Medical Publications.

Ryan, J. F. (1972) 'I.Q. The illusion of objectivity' in K. Richardson and D. Spears (eds) *Race, Culture and Intelligence* London, Penguin.

Ryan, J. (1975) 'The language of stupidity' in J. Morton (ed.) *The Language of Stupidity* London, Elek.

Ryle, G. (1948) *The Concept of Mind* London, Hutchinson.

Schatzman, L. and Strauss, A. (1966) 'A sociology of psychiatry, a perspective and some organising foci' *Social Problems* 14, p. 3.

Scheff, T. (1963) 'Decision rules and types of error in medical diagnosis' *Behavioural Science* 8, p. 97.

Scheff, T. J. (1966) *Being Mentally Ill* London, Weidenfeld and Nicolson.

Scheff, T. (1968) 'Negotiating reality, notes on power in the assessment of responsibility' *Social Problems* 16, p. 3.

Schegloff, E. and Sacks, H. (1973) 'Opening up closings' *Semiotica* 3, p. 4.

Schutz, A. (1962) *Collected Papers Vol. I. The Problem of Social Reality* The Hague, Martinus Nijhoff.

Schutz, A. (1970) *Reflections on the Problem of Relevance* R. M. Zaner (ed.) New Haven, Conn., Yale University Press.

Schutz, A. and Luckman, T. (1974) *The Structures of the Life-World* London, Heinemann.

Scott, M. and Lyman, S. (1968) 'Accounts' *American Sociological Review* 33, p. 46.

Sedgewick, P. (1973) 'Mental illness *is* illness' *Salmagundi* 20, p. 196.

Sharaf, M. and Levinson, D. (1964) 'The quest for omnipotence in professional training' *Psychiatry* 27, p. 135.

Siegel, E. and Dillehay, R. C. (1966) 'Some approaches to family planning counselling in local health departments' *Amer. J. Publ. Hlth.* 56, p. 1840.

Siirala, M. (1969) *Medicine in Metamorphosis* London, Tavistock Publications.

Siirala, M. (1972) 'Psychotherapy of schizophrenia as basic human experience' *Psychiatra Fennica* 155, Yearbook of the Psychiatric Clinic of the Helsinki University Central Hospital.

Siirala, M. (1975) 'Anthropological structure of depression' *The Human Context* 7, p. 530.

Simar, A. and Boyer, E. G. (1968) 'Mirrors for behaviour' *Classroom Interaction. Newsletter* 3, p. 2.

Sinclair, J. McH. and Coulthard, R. M. (1964) *Beginning the Analysis of Discourse: The Language Used by Teachers and Pupils* London, Oxford University Press.

Smith, H. L. (1957) 'Psychiatry in medicine' *American Journal of Sociology* 63, p. 285.

Stein, L. I. (1968) 'The doctor—nurse game' *Amer. J. of Nursing* 68, p. 101.

Stimson, G. V. (1974) 'Obeying doctor's orders: a view from the other side' *Soc. Sci. & Med.* 8, p. 97.

Stimson, G. and Webb, B. (1975) *Going to see the Doctor: the consultation process in general practice* London, Routledge & Kegan Paul.

Stoetzel, J. (1960) 'La maladie, le malade et le medecin' *Population* 12, p. 613.

Strauss, A. L. *et al.* (1964) *Psychiatric Ideologies and Institutions* Glencoe, Ill., Free Press.

Susser, M. W. (1973) *Causal Thinking in the Health Sciences* Oxford, University Press.

Szasz, T. (1960) 'The myth of mental illness' *American Psychologist* 15, p. 113.

Szasz, T. (1970) *The Manufacture of Madness* New York, Harper and Row.

Tait, I. (1973) 'Behavioural science in medical education and clinical practice' *Soc. Sci. and Med.* 7, p. 1003.

Tanner, T. (1969) 'Introduction to Jane Austen' *Sense and Sensibility* Harmondsworth, Penguin Books.

Taylor, I., Walton, P. and Young, J. (1973) *The New Criminology* London, Routledge & Kegan Paul.

Tew, B. J. (1973) 'Some psychological consequences of spina bifida and its complications' *Proceedings of the 31st Biennial Conference* London, Association for Special Education.

Voysey, M. (1972a) 'Impression management by parents of the disabled: the reconstruction of good parents' *J. Health and Soc. Behav.* 13, p. 80.

Voysey, M. (1972b) 'Official agents and the legitimation of suffering' *Sociol. Rev.* 20, p. 533.

Wadsworth, M. E. J. (1974) 'Health and sickness' *J. psychosom. res.* 18, p. 271.

Wagner, H. R. (1970) *Alfred Schutz: On Phenomenology and Social Relations* Chicago, University Press.

Walker, J. H., Thomas, M. and Russell, I. T. (1971) 'Spina bifida — and the parents' *Devel. Med. and Child Neurol.* 13, p. 462.

Wellman, B. (1969) 'On negotiating reality' *Social Problems* 16, p. 537.

Werthman, C. (1968) 'Delinquency and moral character' in Donald R. Cressey and David A. Ward (eds) *Delinquency, Crime and Social Process* London, Harper and Row.

Williams, R. (1965) *The Long Revolution* Harmondsworth, Pelican.

Wilson, W. (1970) 'Social psychology and mental retardation' in N. R. Ellis (ed.) *International Review of Research in Mental Retardation* (vol. 4) New York, Academic Press.

Wittgenstein, L. (1961) *Tractatus logico-philosophicus* London, Routledge & Kegan Paul.

Wittgenstein, L. (1972) *Philosophical Investigations* Oxford, Blackwell.

Wynne, L. C., Ryckoff, I., Day, J. and Hirsch, S. (1958) 'Pseudo-mutuality in the family relations of schizophrenics' *Psychiatry, Journal for the Study of Interpersonal Processes* 21, p. 205.

Younghusband, E., Birchall, D., Davie, R. and Pringle, M. L. K. (eds) (1970) *Living with Handicap* London, National Bureau for Co-operation in Child Care.

Zigler, E. (1967) 'Familial retardation — a continuing dilemma' *Science* 155, p. 292.

Zimmerman, D. H. and Wieder, D. L. (1971) 'Ethnomethodology and the problem of order' in J. D. Douglas *Understanding Everyday Life* London, Routledge & Kegan Paul.

Zola, I. K. (1972) 'Medicine as an institution of social control' *Soc. Rev.* 20, p. 487.